Perkins and Hansell's
Atlas of Diseases of the Eye

For Churchill Livingstone

Publisher: Michael Parkinson
Project Editor: Dilys Jones
Copy Editor: Andrew Gardiner
Production Controller: Debra Barrie
Design: Design Resources Unit
Sales Promotion Executive: Duncan Jones

Perkins and Hansell's Atlas of Diseases of the Eye

91 328

Damian O'Neill, FRCS FCOphth MRCP(I) DO

Registrar, Moorfields Eye Hospital, London

FOURTH EDITION

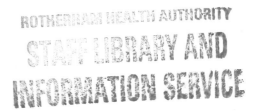

CHURCHILL LIVINGSTONE
EDINBURGH LONDON MADRID MELBOURNE NEW YORK AND TOKYO 1994

CHURCHILL LIVINGSTONE
Medical Division of Longman Group UK Limited

Distributed in the United States of America by Churchill
Livingstone Inc., 650 Avenue of the Americas, New York, N.Y.
10011, and by associated companies, branches and
representatives throughout the world.

First edition 1957
Second edition 1971
Third edition 1986
Fourth edition 1994

ISBN 0-443-04822-3

British Library of Cataloguing in Publication Data
A catalogue record for this book is available from the British Library.

Library of Congress Cataloging in Publication Data
O'Neill, Damian.
    Perkins and Hansell's atlas of diseases of the eye/Damian
O'Neill. -- 4th ed.
        p.   cm.
    Includes index.
    Rev. ed. of: An atlas of diseases of the eye/E.S. Perkins, Peter
Hansell, Ronald J. Marsh. 3rd ed. 1986.
    ISBN 0-443-04822-3
    1. Eye--Diseases and defects--Atlases. 2. Ophthalmology--Atlases.
  I. Perkins, Edward S. (Edward Sylvester). Atlas of diseases of the
    eye. II. Hansell, Peter. III. Title. IV. Title: Atlas of diseases
    of the eye.
    [DNLM: 1. Opthalmology--atlases. 2. Eye Diseases--atlases. WW
17 058p 1993]
RE71.P38 1993
617.7'00022'2--dc20
DNLM/DLC
for Library of Congress   93-9993
                                                               CIP

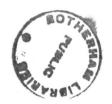

Printed in Hong Kong
LYP/01

Contents

Preface to the Fourth Edition

The purpose of this book remains unchanged, namely, to provide the student, the general medical practitioner and specialists in other branches of medicine with an easily assimilable illustrated guide to the more common and important ocular disorders. It is not intended as a comprehensive atlas for the ophthalmologist, as this need is served by other publications, but it is hoped that residents commencing ophthalmic training will find the work useful as an introduction to the subject.

In this new and expanded edition, an effort has been made wherever possible to replace drawings with photographs, but in some instances, particularly in fundus conditions, the static monocular view afforded by the fundus camera does not reveal the more subtle changes that can be accented in a drawing. Every care has been taken to ensure that the text, though brief, is accurate but inevitably, with such rapid advances in

knowledge and the unavoidable lapse of time between manuscript and publication, some small details may already be outdated.

There are additional new chapters dealing with ophthalmic HIV and AIDS, gradual and sudden loss of vision, and the painful red eye. The material which covers the following subjects has been extensively updated and rewritten: cataract surgery, squint, glaucoma, diabetic retinopathy.

There are numerous additional illustrations and the text has been extensively revised and updated.

Finally, the publishers are once again to be congratulated on maintaining the price at an attainable level.

E.S.P.
P.H.
Iowa, Bath and London, 1993
D.O'N.

Acknowledgements

A compilation of this character can never be complete and must inevitably depend upon many sources of material.

Although only a few illustrations from the previous editions have been retained, our collective thanks to the medical staff of Moorfields Eye Hospital and the Institute of Ophthalmology for their initial support must be recorded.

We are pleased to acknowledge more recent and substantial help from the medical illustration services spanning the Institute, Moorfields, the Western Ophthalmic Hospital, the Department of Ophthalmology, University of Iowa and wish to name respectively T. R. Tarrant, R. T. Fletcher, Colin Hood, Miss Susan Ford and Paul Montague in this regard.

The authors wish to thank the following individuals for the use of photographs: Mr J. R. O. Collin for Figs 6.6 and 39.3; Miss E. Graham for Fig. 30.1, Dr A. Hall for Figs 39.1 and 39.2; Mr A. M. P. Hamilton for Fig. 25.1; Mr M. Sanders for Fig. 20.4; and Mr A. D. McG. Steele for Figs 18.11, 18.12, 18.13 and 18.14. Our gratitude is also due to Mr G. Rose, Consultant Ophthalmologist, Moorfields Eye Hospital, for his helpful suggestions.

Copyright for Figs 2.9, 7.4, 17.3, 18.11, 18.12, 18.13, 18.14, 18.15, 20.3, 21.6, 22.2 and 30.5 belongs to Moorfields Eye Hospital, London.

Illustrations

1 The normal eye

Although a detailed knowledge of the normal anatomy of the eye and orbit is not necessary for an understanding of most of the conditions illustrated in this Atlas, some reminder of the gross anatomy and its terminology may be helpful as an introduction.

The eyelids

The eyelids consist essentially of a plate of condensed fibrous tissue (the tarsal plate) lined internally by conjuctiva and covered externally by the orbicularis muscle and skin. The Meibomian glands are embedded in the tarsal plate and open on the free margin of the lid very close to its posterior border.

The palpebral fissure is the almond-shaped space formed when the lids are open. It will be seen from 1.1 and 1.2 that normally the upper lid cuts across the upper part of the cornea, while the lower lid margin is related to the junction between cornea and sclera — the limbus.

The inner and outer angles of the palpebral fissure are known as the inner and outer canthi and at the inner canthus can be seen the caruncle and plica semi-lunaris. On the lid margin by the plica semilunaris is a small elevation known as the papilla lacrimalis in the centre of which is a hole, the punctum lacrimalis, through which the tears flow. The punctum lies in close apposition to the globe and cannot normally be seen unless the lid is everted.

The globe

The eyeball is so positioned in the orbit that the anterior surface of the cornea is just in line with the superior and inferior orbital margins — a useful relation in the assessment of proptosis.

The cornea joins the sclera at the limbus, the corneal epithelium becoming continuous with the epithelium of the conjunctiva which is adherent here to the underlying episcleral tissue. Elsewhere the conjunctiva forms a loose covering for the globe and extends peripherally to form two pockets, the upper and lower fornices, before continuing onto the posterior surface of the lids (1.3).

The anterior chamber is the space enclosed by the cornea anteriorly and the lens and iris posteriorly. The pupillary margin of the iris is in constant contact with the anterior surface of the lens, although aqueous humour is able to flow from the posterior chamber (the small space between the periphery of the iris and the lens) through the pupil into the anterior chamber, from which it drains through the trabeculae into Schlemm's canal.

The iris, ciliary body and choroid form a continuous structure called the uveal tract which is derived embryologically in part from the anterior portion of the optic cup and in part from the surrounding mesoderm.

The choroid is a purely vascular structure which supplies the outer one-third of the retina with blood. 1.3 is a diagrammatic sagittal section through the eye and orbit, showing the gross relations of the bony orbit, lids, globe and intra-ocular structures.

The slit-lamp microscope

Several conditions in this Atlas are illustrated by pictures of slit-lamp appearances and for those unfamiliar with the apparatus a brief description is included here.

The instrument consists of two parts: a low-power binocular microscope mounted horizontally and an illumination system which provides a bright slit of variable width focusing sharply at the point of focus of the microscope. It is designed primarily to examine the transparent media of the eye, i.e. the cornea, aqueous humour, lens and vitreous. The narrow slit beam gives the effect of an optical section in transparent or semitransparent structures and clearly demonstrates differences in optical density due to anatomical structure or pathological change.

As can be seen in the photograph of a normal eye (1.4), the anterior and posterior surfaces of the cornea show clearly, the corneal stroma reflects some light but the normal aqueous humour is optically empty. The anterior surface of the lens shows well and the discontinuity of the layers of the lens substance can be seen.

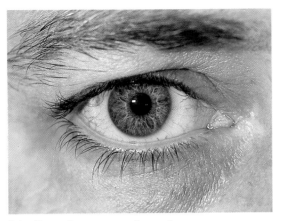

1.1 External appearance of normal eye

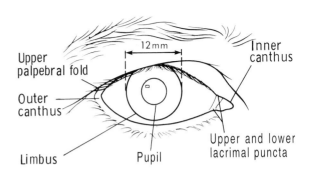

Upper palpebral fold

Outer canthus

Limbus

12mm

Inner canthus

Pupil

Upper and lower lacrimal puncta

1.2 External appearance of normal eye

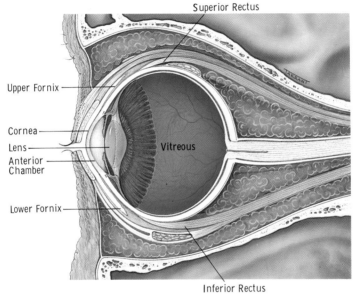

Superior Rectus

Upper Fornix

Cornea

Lens

Anterior Chamber

Vitreous

Lower Fornix

Inferior Rectus

1.3 Sagittal section through orbit

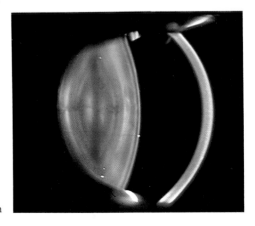

1.4 Eye seen by slit lamp illumination

2 The orbit

The symptoms and signs of orbital disease are protrusion of the globe (proptosis), double vision (diplopia), pain and reduction in vision. The bony walls of the orbit cannot expand easily so that any space-occupying lesion of the orbital contents is likely to cause protrusion of the globe. Inflammations of the orbital tissues, neoplasms of the orbital structures (2.1), or optic nerve and swelling of the soft tissues, particularly the extra-ocular muscles in Graves's disease, are the most common causes of proptosis. The direction of displacement of the globe gives some guide to the position of the lesion. Diplopia may result from limitation of movement of the eye, but it is only in neoplasms of the optic nerve that vision is affected early. Vascular lesions may cause a pulsating exophthalmos and a bruit may be heard over the orbit. Computerized tomography and magnetic resonance imaging (2.2) have greatly improved the non-invasive diagnosis of orbital lesions.

Orbital cellulitis

Extension of infection from the nasal sinuses or skin of the face may involve the orbit, giving rise to acute swelling of the orbital tissues, proptosis and oedema of the conjunctiva and lids (2.3). In children the condition may result from haematogenous spread of infection from a distant site. If untreated there is a risk of the more serious condition of cavernous sinus thrombosis developing and this will usually be accompanied by neurological signs, visual loss, muscle paresis and papilloedema. Meningeal signs may follow and the condition may become bilateral. Treatment with high doses of antibiotic is urgent and attempts should be made to culture the organism from septic lesions on the face, the nose or the cerebrospinal fluid, so that the most suitable drug can be chosen.

Subacute and chronic orbital inflammation may be associated with chronic inflammatory conditions such as sarcoidosis or syphilis and there is also a group of conditions, known as pseudotumour, characterized by non-neoplastic infiltration of the orbital tissue by lymphocytes or plasma cells. Painful proptosis, lid oedema and chemosis are typical signs and all the orbital structures may be involved. Computerised tomography (CT scanning) may demonstrate the diffuse inflammation of orbital structures. The condition responds to systemic corticosteroid therapy.

Mucocele

A mucocele results from chronic infection of one of the paranasal sinuses which becomes blocked and is converted into a fluid filled cyst which enlarges and expands the sinus, frequently encroaching on the orbital cavity and producing proptosis (2.4). Radiography will show enlargement of the sinus with erosion of the bony wall of the orbit. Treatment is by surgical removal of the cyst and re-establishment of drainage into the nose.

Tumours of orbit

Benign tumours arise from a large number of tissues in the orbit and include: dermoid cysts (2.5), fibrous histiocytomas, haemangioma (2.6), glioma, meningioma, neuroma and haemangiopericytoma.

Primary malignant tumours are unusual in the orbit but include lacrimal carcinoma, malignant fibrous histiocytoma, haemangioma, embryonal sarcoma and rhabdomyosarcoma. Malignant changes can occur in haemangiomas, bony tumours or dermoids (2.5). Malignant diseases of blood and lymphoid systems, in particular leukaemia, may present with infiltration of the orbit. Finally, metastases can occur in the orbit and in young children; these tend to derive from the kidney and adrenal gland. The commonest sources of orbital metastases in the adult are primary tumours of the breast or bronchus.

Diagnosis of orbital tumours is made by considering the direction of displacement of the globe by general examination of the patient, X-rays, CT scan, ultrasound and orbital venography. Orbital biopsy may be necessary in some cases. Benign tumours and some of the less malignant tumours may be completely removed by lateral orbitotomy.

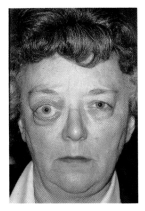

2.1 Tumour of the orbit

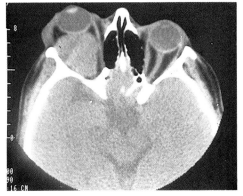

2.2 CT scan picture showing orbital tumour

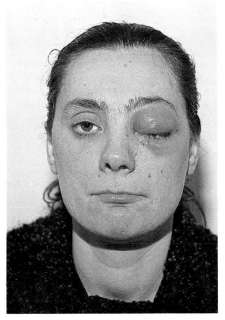

2.3 Orbital cellulitis

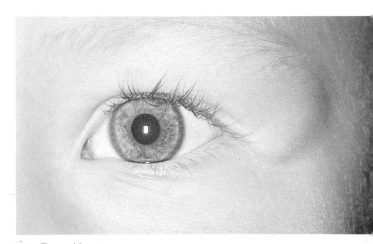

2.5 Dermoid cyst

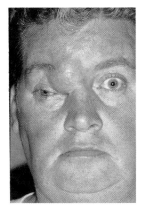

2.4 Mucocele

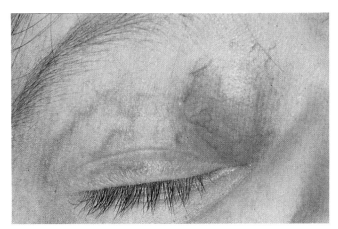

2.6 Haemangioma

2 The orbit (cont.)

Endocrine exophthalmos

The association between disease of the thyroid gland and exophthalmos has been recognized for over 100 years, but although the clinical picture is so characteristic, the underlying pathology is still not clear. Briefly, two syndromes can be distinguished: first, a slight exophthalmos with marked lid retraction occurring in thyrotoxicosis, and secondly, a more severe proptosis associated with ophthalmoplegia, which may follow thyroidectomy or may occur *ab initio* in patients with normal or subnormal thyroid activity.

The staring appearance of patients with thyrotoxicosis is so well known as to require little description except to emphasize that the actual protrusion of the eyes is usually small and the appearance is largely due to the lid retraction. 2.7 is a photograph of such a patient, showing how the upper lid is raised to expose the sclera above the cornea. In the majority of cases the ocular condition improves when the thyroid overactivity has been reduced either by medical or surgical treatment. Any remaining disfigurement can be overcome by a small lateral tarsorrhaphy or operations to weaken the retractor muscles of the eyelids.

The cardinal feature of the more serious exophthalmos associated with thyroid disease is the involvement of the extra-ocular muscles. These become thickened and swollen by a lymphocytic infiltration and deposition of mucopolysaccharides and collagen. Proptosis, which initially may be unilateral is followed by limitation of movement of the globe, chemosis, damage to the cornea due to exposure and, in some cases, visual loss resulting from compression of the optic nerve by the swollen muscle bellies in the apex of the orbit (2.8). The important role of the extra-ocular muscles is reflected in the name Graves' ophthalmopathy which is now frequently used for this condition. CT scanning is a particularly useful procedure for identifying muscle swelling in dysthyroid ophthalmopathy (Graves' disease) (2.9).

The initial treatment of exophthalmos in dysthyroid eye disease is directed to protection of the cornea and relief of the pressure on the optic nerve. High dose steroid therapy, surgical orbital decompression or orbital radiotherapy may be necessary in severe cases. When the condition has stabilized operations on the extra-ocular muscles can improve the field of binocular single vision and reduce the diplopia caused by limitation of movement of the globe.

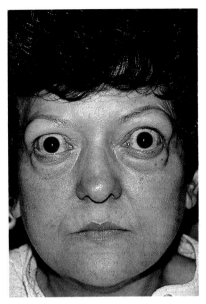

2.7 Thyrotoxicosis

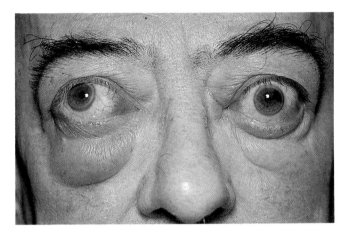

2.8 Thyrotropic exophthalmos

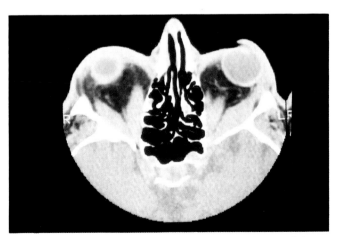

2.9 CT scan showing rectus muscle enlargement and proptosis in
dysthyroid eye disease

3 *The lids*

Ptosis

A drooping lid on one or both sides is a common congenital defect. The degree of ptosis varies from a hardly perceptible narrowing of the palpebral fissure to a complete paralysis of elevation of the upper lid, which hangs down obscuring the pupil (3.1). The patient attempts to remedy the condition by raising the eyebrow, by contracting the frontalis muscle and tilting the head back, producing a very typical appearance. The absence or weakness of the levator palpebrae superioris muscle, which is the cause of the ptosis, may be associated with weakness or absence of the superior rectus muscle. Acquired ptosis is usually due to age-related degenerative changes in the levator palpebrae superioris muscle and its tendon. Acquired ptosis may also be the presenting feature of neurologic or muscular disorders such as myaesthenia gravis, myopathies. Horner's syndrome, or oculomotor nerve palsy.

Epicanthus

The term epicanthus is used to describe the vertical skin folds at the inner canthi, seen in the photograph (3.2). Such folds are normal during foetal development from the third to the sixth month but, in the Caucasian races, they have normally disappeared by birth. In the Mongolian races, on the other hand, the condition persists into adult life, giving rise to the typical Mongolian eye. When it persists in the Caucasian races the child is seen to have a broad flat nose with widely separated eyes and often an apparent convergent squint. Careful examination, however, will show that the eyes are actually straight and the epicanthal folds and the apparent squint can frequently be made to disappear by pinching up the loose skin over the bridge of the nose. Many mild cases cure themselves when the nose develops normally at puberty or before. In more severe cases operative procedures are necessary.

Ectropion

This is a condition in which the lower lid falls away from the globe and becomes everted. The drainage of tears takes place mainly through the lower punctum and unless this is in close apposition to the globe it is unable to function and epiphora results. The constant flow of tears over the lid, combined with wiping the eye with a handkerchief, causes excoriation and subsequent retraction of the skin, tending to aggravate the eversion.

Ectropion may be caused by scarring of the skin, as for example following irradiation of a rodent ulcer, or more commonly through a lessening of muscle tone combined with a decrease in orbital fat in old people which allows the lower lid to fall away from the globe. There may be a spastic element present also — the lower fibres of the orbicularis muscle contracting more than the fibres near the lid margin, thus tending to cause eversion of the lid.

3.3 is a photograph of typical senile ectropion. The conjunctival surface of the lid is exposed and the punctum is well away from the globe. The skin at the inner canthus is excoriated and taut, pulling the lid downwards. The exposed conjunctiva becomes chronically inflamed and unsightly. Usually some plastic procedure is necessary to bring the lid back into its normal position.

Entropion

In entropion the lid turns inwards and the lashes cause much irritation by rubbing on the cornea. Unlike ectropion it may affect either the upper or lower lid. Again the causes are scarring, this time of the tarsal plate, and senile changes of muscle tone in which the marginal fibres of the orbicularis contract more strongly than the peripheral fibres, thus turning the lid inwards. The latter condition of senile spastic entropion is much more common in this country than the cicatricial entropion of the upper lid following such diseases as trachoma, in which the tarsal plate is severely scarred and buckled.

Spastic entropion is only present intermittently at first but can be elicited by asking the patient to squeeze the eyes tightly shut, when, on subsequent opening, the lower lid will be seen to be turned inwards. This is well shown in 3.5. A slight pull on the skin of the lid will replace it in its normal position. After a while the lid becomes inverted more frequently and corneal ulceration from the abrasions caused by the lashes may result. Treatment consists of operative procedures designed to strengthen the lower fibres of the orbicularis or weaken the marginal fibres. 3.4 shows an upper lid entropion caused by scarring and contracture of the conjunctiva.

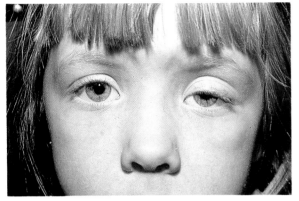

3.1 Ptosis

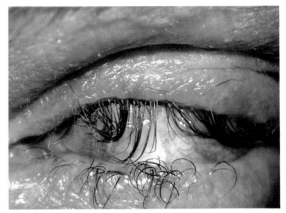

3.2 Epicanthus

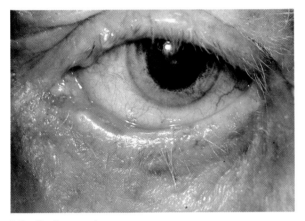

3.3 Senile ectropion

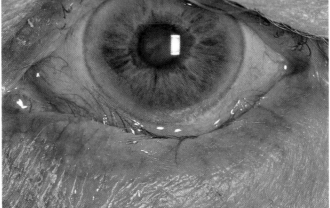

3.4 Cicatricial entropion of upper eyelid

3.5 Spastic entropion

4 The lids: inflammatory lesions

Marginal cysts

The glands of Moll are sweat glands occurring in the lid margin associated with the lashes, and not uncommonly they become blocked to form cystic swellings. These have a predilection for the lower lid near the lacrimal punctum as illustrated in 4.1.

Sebaceous cysts occur in the lids as elsewhere in the skin. They may arise from the glands of Zeis, which are sebaceous glands associated with the lashes, producing a similar appearance to the sweat gland cyst illustrated in 4.1. These should be referred for excision because of the proximity of the lacrimal punctum.

Blepharitis

Chronic inflammation of the lid margins is a very common and distressing condition. The inflammation may be mild and consist simply in a hyperaemia of the lid margin with scaling of the skin (squamous blepharitis) or may be more severe and affect the lash follicles, leading to destruction or distortion of the lashes and deformity of the lid margin (ulcerative blepharitis).

Both types are commonly associated with seborrhoea of the skin. 4.2 shows a long-standing case of ulcerative blepharitis in which the lid margins are deformed, many lashes are missing and others are distorted and turn in to rub on the cornea. Blepharitis is a chronic condition with periodic exacerbations. It is not possible to cure blepharitis although symptoms can be alleviated by a number of mechanical and medical measures. Mechanical treatments include regular lid toilet (wiping crusts and scales from the lid margin) as well as surgical correction of any malposition of the lid margin or eyelashes (entropion, ectropion or trichiasis).

Topical antibiotics are prescribed in short courses for secondary conjunctivitis and systemic tetracyclines may be used for several months to treat inflammation of the lid Meibomian glands. Topical lubricants such as hypromellose eye drops may be used to alleviate symptoms.

Hordeolum or stye

This well known and common condition is essentially a staphylococcal infection of a lash follicle and corresponds to a boil of the skin elsewhere. It starts as a painful swelling of the whole lid so that at first it may be difficult to find a localized lesion, but soon one area becomes more swollen and, as pus forms, a yellow point associated with an eyelash can be seen near the lid margin (4.3).

The differential diagnosis is from an acute inflammation of the Meibomian glands — the so-called hordeolum internum. A stye is in the skin and always associated with the lashes, while a Meibomian infection is in the tarsal plate and the skin is not primarily involved. Examination of the conjunctival surface of the lid in hordeolum internum will show a red velvety area with a central yellow spot, through which pus will later discharge. As the Meibomian glands are embedded in tough fibrous tissue, pain and reaction may be more severe than in an ordinary stye.

Local treatment is by heat until the abscess points, when it may be opened to allow drainage of the pus. Removal of the affected lash is frequently sufficient in a hordeolum externum.

Chalazion

This is a chronic affection of the Meibomian glands. A painless firm lump appears in the lid and slowly increases in size (4.4). Frequently called a Meibomian cyst, it is, however, not truly cystic but a chronic granuloma caused primarily by the retention of the secretion of the gland. The skin moves freely over the swelling and if the lid is everted a grey spot surrounded by inflamed conjunctiva will be seen at the site of the lesion. Treatment is incision and curettage through the conjunctival surface of the lid. Some chalazia disappear spontaneously. Persistent or uncomfortable chalazia can be incised and curetted from the conjunctival surface.

Molluscum contagiosum

Molluscum contagiosum is a virus disease producing small umbilicated pimples on the skin of the lids (4.5). The lesions tend to spread and cause a secondary conjunctivitis, often follicular in type. If the condition is left untreated a superficial keratitis may develop. The lesions on the skin should be incised and the contents squeezed out.

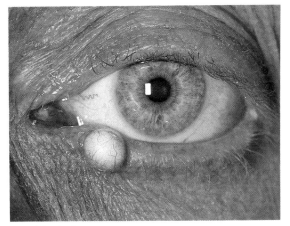

4.1 Marginal cyst

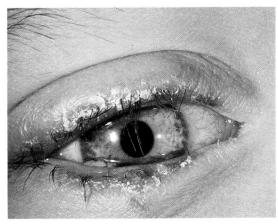

4.2 Ulcerative blepharitis

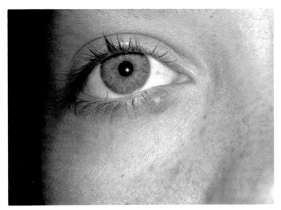

4.3 Stye

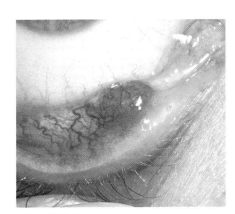

4.4 Chalazion

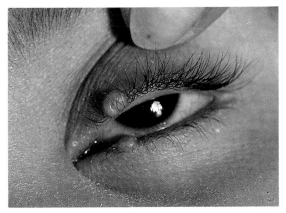

4.5 Molluscum contagiosum

5 *The lids: skin conditions*

Almost any skin condition may affect the lids but only those in which the region of the eyelids is primarily involved or which have particular ocular significance will be discussed and illustrated here.

Contact dermatitis

This very common condition may follow the topical application of drugs, cosmetics or any foreign material. It is of particular importance in ophthalmology, in which the continued use of drops and ointments frequently causes an allergic reaction in a sensitive patient. Penicillin ointment applied to the lids, and atropine drops, very commonly cause such irritation.

The changes in the skin are essentially eczematous in nature and usually arise after repeated use of the agent. Itching is a prominent symptom and the skin of the lids, particularly the lower lid, becomes red and scaly, and in severe cases the inflammation may spread over the whole face.

5.1 illustrates a case of contact dermatitis following the use of eye drops. The lids are swollen and the skin shows vesiculation extending well beyond the lids, an appearance which always suggests a drug reaction. Treatment includes avoiding substances known to precipitate dermatitis in a given patient. Secondary skin infection is treated with appropriate antibiotic or antifungal drugs, though this complication is uncommon. Topical steroid may be used in short courses at low concentration. Prolonged topical steroid use causes thinning of the lid skin.

Oedema of the lids

The thin skin and loose subcutaneous tissue of the lids predispose to oedema in this region. Local inflammations, angioneurotic oedema, renal disease, myxoedema and parasitic infestation with trypanosomiasis and trichiniasis (in which marked swelling of the lids is an important symptom) are some of the many causes.

In myxoedema the swelling is not a true oedema and does not pit on pressure. The puffy lids with the dry skin and sparse eyebrows help to give the characteristic facies of the disease. An advanced case is illustrated in 5.2. In this patient the left eye is severely affected and ptosis has resulted from the swelling and weight of the upper lid.

Xanthelasma

The skin of the lids, particularly towards the inner canthus, is a common site for the deposition of lipid material. 5.3 shows the typical yellowish, soft plaques. Xanthelasma affects women more frequently than men and it may be associated with a hyperlipaemia. It causes no symptoms but may require excision for cosmetic reasons.

Acne rosacea

This common skin disease is frequently associated with a blepharo-conjunctivitis and sometimes a keratitis. The typical flushing of the skin of the cheeks (5.4) often extends to the lids, causing a scaly desquamation and diffuse hyperaemia. The conjunctiva shows engorgement of the vessels with some hypersecretion. The condition is not serious unless or until the cornea is affected. The facial rash can be treated with oral tetracycline or erythromycin over several months. Topical 1% ichthyol in zinc or 2% aqueous sulphur cream are also effective. There is a high relapse rate once topical antibiotics or topical creams are stopped.

Herpes ophthalmicus

Herpes zoster involving the ophthalmic division of the trigeminal nerve is of particular importance because of the ocular complications. The history of onset with pain and constitutional disturbance followed by erythema and vesicle formation is characteristic. The lesions may occur in the area of distribution of the whole of the ophthalmic division of the trigeminal nerve or a part only. The frontal branch is always involved but it is when the lacrimal and nasociliary branches are also affected that corneal involvement and iritis are likely to occur. It is a good working rule that if the side of the tip of the nose is involved, eye complications are likely. Similarly all patients with decreased vision or photophobia should be suspected of having viral keratitis or uveitis and referred for specialist opinion. 5.5 shows the typical distribution and appearance of the vesicles. The frontal branch of the trigeminal nerve is mainly affected in this case.

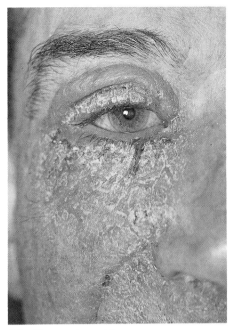

5.1 Contact dermatitis

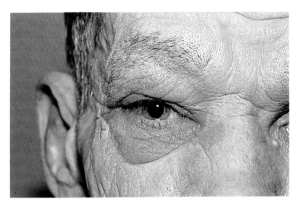

5.2 Localised myxoedema

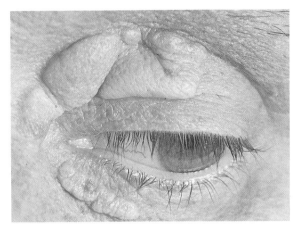

5.3 Xanthelasma

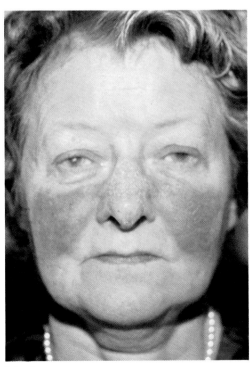

5.4 Acne rosacea

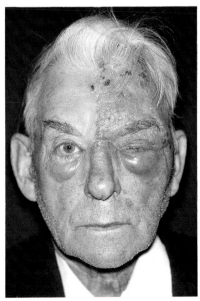

5.5 Herpes ophthalmicus

6 *The lids: neoplasms*

Epidermal papilloma

Papillomas occur along the lid margin and are often multiple; they may be found in children but are more frequent in people over middle age. They are benign and can be excised for cosmetic reasons (6.1).

Pre-cancerous lesions include: actinic keratoses, Bowen's disease and xeroderma pigmentosum. Treatment is local excision.

Malignant neoplasms

The lids and skin of the nose near the inner canthus are very common sites for the development of carcinoma in older people. Basal cell carcinomas or rodent ulcers are more common than squamous epitheliomas and are characterized histologically by downgrowths of solid darkly staining cells into the dermis. Clinically a rodent ulcer starts as a small nodule in the skin which gradually enlarges and breaks down to form an ulcer with indurated base and rolled edges. Bleeding from the ulcer is common but any skin nodule which has been present for several months in a patient over the age of 40 should be viewed with suspicion. A small wedge-shaped biopsy may be taken to confirm the diagnosis. Early removal may save the otherwise inevitable growth of the tumour with much destruction of the lid tissues. Radiation may be preferable but special precautions must be taken to avoid damage to the globe

itself. Where the tumour overlies the lacrimal drainage apparatus it is preferable to carry out local excision. 6.2 is a photograph of a typical basal cell carcinoma of the lid. The rolled edges and breaking down base of the ulcer can be clearly seen. Squamous cell carcinoma is less common than rodent ulcer but tends to be more malignant and may metastasise to lymph nodes in the preauricular or submaxillary region. Histologically the tumour shows more resemblance to the general structure of the epidermis. Well developed prickle cells surround areas of squamous cells which undergo their normal degeneration to form cell nests of acid staining cornified epithelial cells. Clinically it appears either as an ulcerated area less symmetrical than a rodent ulcer or as a papillomatous growth. Local extension occurs slowly but relentlessly eating away the lids, the soft structures of the orbit and even the bone itself if the tumour is left untreated. 6.3 shows a squamous cell carcinoma which has destroyed a considerable amount of the tissue of the lower lid; in such cases plastic surgery is required to fill in the defect after excision of the growth. Particular care should be taken to remove the whole of the tumour as the mortality rate is appreciable. Careful follow-up examination is necessary for many years.

Tumours of sweat glands and sebaceous glands are rare.

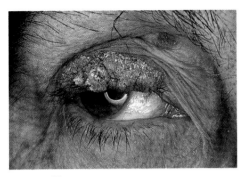

6.1 Papilloma

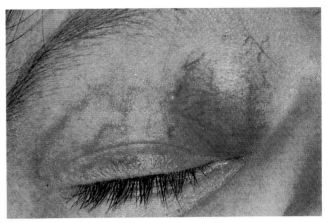

6.4 Cavernous haemangioma

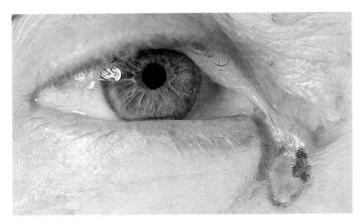

6.2 Basal cell carcinoma

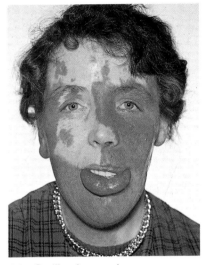

6.5 Capillary haemangioma

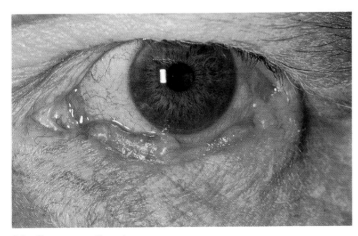

6.3 Squamous cell carcinoma

Melanogenic system

Naevi may occur on the lids, rarely they become malignant and require generous surgical removal.

Vascular tumours

These are generally benign and include capillary, cavernous and racemose haemangiomata and lymphangioma. The cavernous are relatively common congenital lesions of the lids giving rise to bluish soft swellings which can be reduced by pressure (6.4). They tend to enlarge in the first few years of life and may, if they involve the orbit, cause ptosis or exophthalmos. Capillary haemangiomata — the typical port wine stains — are more common and of particular interest as they may be associated with meningeal and choroidal lesions (the Sturge-Weber syndrome (6.5)). Associated structural anomalies in the anterior segment of the eye are common with congenital or infantile glaucoma. Sometimes the glaucoma is delayed until adult life.

Argon laser treatment is currently being tried to reduce the haemangioma. It appears that its effects are best in late adolescence and in the darker coloured lesions.

Kaposi's sarcoma

Kaposi's sarcoma is now accepted as a criterion of AIDS in HIV positive individuals. Ocular Kaposi's sarcoma presents as a purple, red or brown macule which slowly progresses to a mass lesion. It can be treated by local surgery, irradiation or intra-lesional chemotherapy (6.6).

Neurofibroma

In neurofibromatosis or von Recklinghausen's disease multiple developmental tumours arise from the sheaths of peripheral nerves. The lids, especially the upper may be involved giving rise to gross enlargement. Such plexiform neuromas may penetrate into the orbit. 6.7 shows a massive lesion of this type.

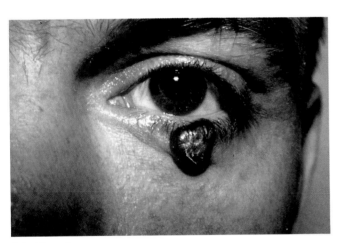

6.6 Kaposi's sarcoma

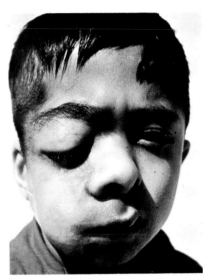

6.7 Neurofibromatosis

7 The lacrimal system

The lacrimal gland

Dacryo-adenitis: acute dacryo-adenitis is rare but may occur as a complication of viral infections including mumps and herpes simplex. A painful swelling appears in the outer region of the upper lid causing some degree of ptosis. On raising the lid the swollen palpebral portion of the gland can be seen bulging under the conjunctiva (7.1).

Chronic enlargement of the lacrimal gland may occur in sarcoidosis (sometimes with uveitis and involvement of the parotid gland) or other inflammatory and tumour-like lesions — so called inflammatory pseudotumours. In this group will be found Mikulicz's syndrome where there is bilateral symmetrical enlargement of the lacrimal and salivary glands due to sarcoidosis, leukaemia, lymphomas, etc.

Lacrimal gland tumours

1. Benign epithelial tumours include pleomorphic adenoma (benign mixed tumour) and mucoepidermoid. The isolated tumours cause painless enlargement of the gland with displacement of the eye forwards, downwards and inwards.
2. Malignant tumours consist of carcinomatous change in the benign mixed cell, adenoid cystic carcinoma and adenocarcinoma tumours (7.2). The prognosis with all of these is poor and treatment is radical excision through a lateral orbitotomy. They are poorly radiosensitive.
3. Haematopoietic or lymphoid tumours occur here and may be localised or associated with systemic disease.

Lacrimal drainage apparatus

Dacryocystitis is generally the result of an obstruction of drainage of the naso-lacrimal duct. It occurs chiefly in babies and females in their 50s and the site of the obstruction is generally at the entrance to the nose. The symptoms are epiphora, swelling and redness at the inner canthus of the eye (7.3). Treatment consists of local hot bathing, antibiotic drops and systemic antibiotics. Spontaneous resolution generally occurs in babies by the age of 1 year. Persistent epiphora in babies after this age should be investigated and treated by diagnostic and therapeutic probing of the lacrimal system under general anaesthesia. The anatomy of the lacrimal drainage system can be investigated by syringing and probing (under topical anaesthesia in adults), and by demonstrating the drainage system radiographically with contrast medium (dacryocystogram) (7.4). Recurrent attacks of dacryocystitis or the formation of a mucoele in adults may necessitate a dacryocystorhinostomy to relieve the obstruction.

Rarely the streptothrix filamentary bacterium may invade the lacrimal drainage system causing chronic inflammation and formation of a large concretion (7.5). Treatment is by opening up the affected cannaliculus, expressing and curetting the contents. Penicillin drops help to cut down the inflammatory response.

Tumours of the lacrimal drainage apparatus are rare and usually epithelial, either benign papillomas or squamous cell, transitional or adenocarcinoma.

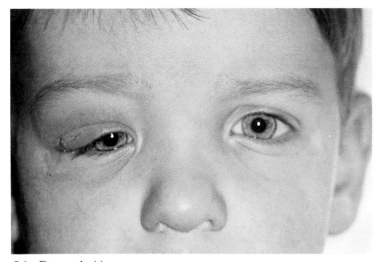

7.1 Dacryoadenitis

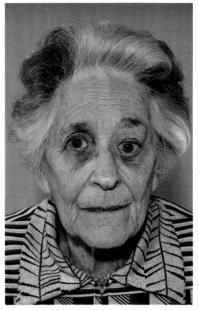

7.2 Malignant tumour of the left lacrimal gland

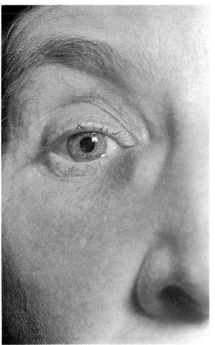

7.3 Acute dacryocystitis

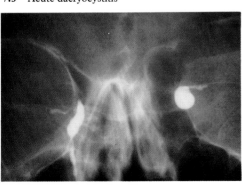

7.4 Dacryocystogram showing blockage of left naso-lacrimal duct

7.5 Canaliculitis

8 *The conjunctiva: inflammations*

The differential diagnosis of a 'red eye' is a common clinical problem and it is usual to divide the type of injection into conjunctival or ciliary. By this is meant that when the vessels supplying the conjunctiva only are dilated the redness is superficial and more marked towards the fornices, but when the deeper vessels which enter the eye to supply the cornea and ciliary body are dilated the redness is less bright in colour and is situated particularly in the limbal area surrounding the cornea. The distinction between the two types of injection is not as clear-cut as is sometimes suggested, but, as demonstrated in 8.1, the majority of cases of simple conjunctivitis show the typical 'conjunctival' type of injection. Not infrequently, however, a conjunctival inflammation is associated with a superficial keratitis and in these cases the injection will always extend to the limbal vessels (8.2).

Acute bacterial conjunctivitis
Acute infective conjunctivitis as illustrated in 8.1 may be caused by a variety of microorganisms and is characterised by a gritty sensation, conjunctival injection and purulent discharge.

Appropriate topical antibiotics should be prescribed. These help prevent keratitis and conjunctival scarring. Neonatal conjunctivitis should be carefully investigated to identify gonococcal and chlamydial infections. All infected patients should be advised about general hygiene measures to avoid cross infection (such as not swimming in public baths and not sharing face towels).

Vernal conjunctivitis
Vernal conjunctivitis is a bilateral recurrent allergic condition with a seasonal incidence, causing itching and redness of the eyes with lacrimation and some mucous discharge.

The papules, well illustrated in 8.3, occur most commonly on the tarsal conjunctiva but there is a more serious group of cases in which the conjunctiva at the limbus is involved, the lesions spreading onto the cornea, which may become completely covered. Sodium cromoglycate and corticosteroid drops can relieve symptoms in most cases.

Phlyctenular conjunctivitis
Phlyctenular conjunctivitis is another type of allergic response by the conjunctiva to an irritant — this time an endogenous agent, typically tuberculo-protein, although other bacterial proteins may have the same effect. It is essentially a disease of children living in overcrowded, unhygienic surroundings on an inadequate diet.

The phlyctens are raised whitish nodules usually occurring near the limbus and accompanied by a leash of dilated conjunctival vessels (8.4). The nodule tends to ulcerate and finally to disappear, only to be succeeded by a similar lesion at another site.

The symptoms of phlyctenular conjunctivitis are usually slight but once the cornea is involved pain, lacrimation and photophobia are marked and it may be very difficult to persuade the child to open the lids sufficiently for the eye to be examined.

The treatment is directed to improving the general health, combined with local steroid therapy.

Chronic conjunctivitis
Chronic conjunctival irritation, causing a gritty feeling, with hyperaemia and a slight mucoid discharge, is a common condition often posing difficulties in aetiological diagnosis. Often there is an infective element such as a chronic blepharitis (Ch. 4); allergy to cosmetics is sometimes responsible and drug intolerance is a common cause, particularly over-treatment with topical antibiotics (Ch. 5). An unsuspected foreign body or exogenous irritants such as chemical fumes or insecticide powders must be considered. Deficiency of lacrimal secretion can also cause similar symptoms (Ch. 13).

Treatment must be directed to the cause if this can be found, and antibiotics or steroid drugs avoided unless there is a clear indication for their use.

Giant papillary conjunctivitis
This condition occurs in some individuals after prolonged use of contact lenses and seems to be more common in those using soft lenses. Papules develop in the conjunctiva of the upper lid and produce symptoms of irritation and mucous discharge. Cleaning deposits off the lens or changing the lens is often effective in reducing the symptoms (8.5).

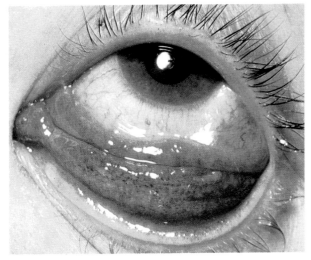

8.1 Acute conjunctivitis

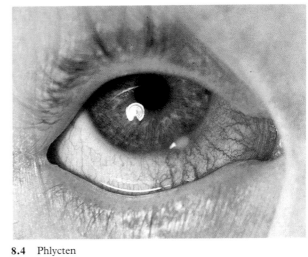

8.4 Phlycten

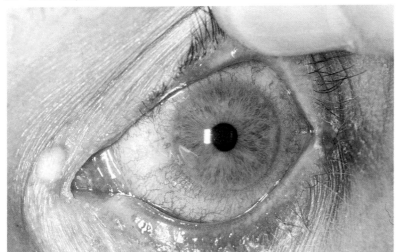

8.2 Keratoconjunctivitis

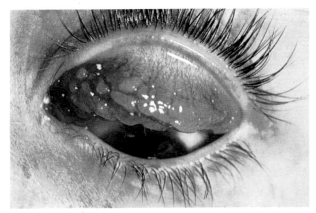

8.3 Vernal conjunctivitis

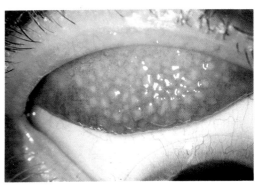

8.5 Contact lens reaction

9 *Viral conjunctivitis*

Viral disease is an important cause of conjunctivitis nowadays. A typical reaction in the conjunctiva to virus is a follicular conjunctivis with a superficial punctate keratitis and frequently enlargement of pre-auricular lymph nodes.

Adenovirus

There are many subtypes of adenovirus. The commonest two are those which cause pharyngoconjunctival fever and epidemic keratoconjunctivitis. Both are highly contagious, the latter frequently occurring in schools and hospitals. The onset is acute with injection, follicle formation, painless pre-auricular lymphadenopathy and is usually bilateral. Rarely subconjunctival haemorrhages are produced and sometimes a pseudomembrane is deposited on the tarsal conjunctiva (9.1). There is no effective antiviral therapy. Antibiotic drops may be useful to prevent secondary infection.

Herpes simplex

An acute infection can occur with this virus with an acute follicular conjunctivitis and painful swelling of the pre-auricular lymph nodes. It is generally unilateral and there may be small herpetic vesicles formed on the adjacent lids and a superficial punctate keratitis. Treatment with topical antivirals is useful, such as IDU and Ara-A or Acyclovir.

Chlamydia

These are the most important viruses affecting the eye. They belong to the psittacosis-lymphogranulomatrachoma group. They occupy a taxonomic position between bacteria and true viruses and are susceptible to treatment with sulphonamides and tetracyclines. Two eye conditions are recognized: trachoma and paratrachoma. It is probable that only one virus is concerned although different sera types are described. Paratrachoma encompasses inclusion conjunctivitis in the newborn and Tric punctate keratoconjunctivitis. In both types, the infection originates in the genital mucosa and adults generally acquire the disease venereally. Clinically all conditions present with papillary hypertrophy, development of lymphoid follicles, a regional painful pre-auricular lymphadenopathy and punctate epithelial keratitis (9.2). Paratrachoma responds well to antibiotic topical treatment; in particular the tetracyclines. It may be necessary where there is a genital reservoir causing repeated infection to use a course of systemic antibiotic for a period of 6 weeks.

Trachoma is a much more serious infection because of the tendency towards greater scarring of the conjunctiva and the cornea. In the early stages the upper tarsal conjunctiva shows the typical papillary hypertrophy with diffuse infiltration, follicles (9.3) and the cornea shows punctate keratitis with pannus formation above (9.4). The symptoms are pain, lacrimation and photophobia (largely due to the corneal involvement). Later the follicles become more numerous and may spread onto the bulbar conjunctiva. The corneal new vessels and infiltration — trachomatous pannus — progress and are frequently seen in all segments of the cornea although the upper half is most severely affected (9.4). There is progressive scarring of the upper lid, entropion and trichiasis (9.5). Reinfection by the virus is common as is bacterial secondary infection. These contribute to the progressive scarring; in particular of the cornea. It is clear the disease is associated with overcrowded unhygienic environmental conditions in hot dry climates with eye–seeking flies. The prime object of treatment is to improve the social and hygienic conditions in which patients live. Acute infections are treated with the tetracycline group of drugs and the late secondary scarring by plastic surgical procedures to the lids and cornea.

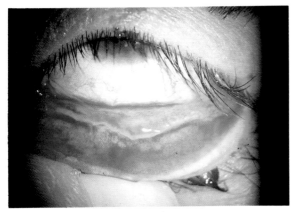

9.1 Pseudomembrane in adenovirus

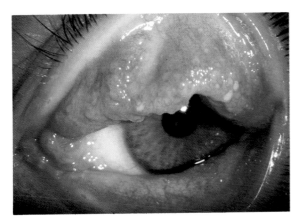

9.2 Follicular conjunctivitis

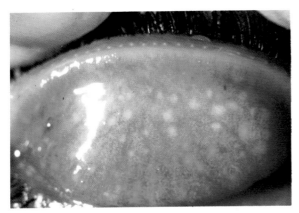

9.3 Trachomatous follicles

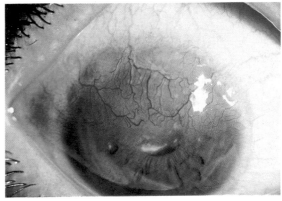

9.4 Trachomatous pannus

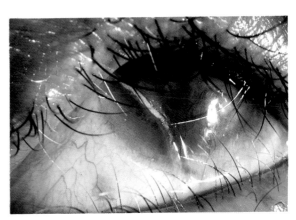

9.5 Trichiasis

10

The conjunctiva: miscellaneous conditions

Subconjunctival haemorrhage

The sudden appearance of an effusion of blood under the conjunctiva is a common happening in an otherwise normal eye. Sometimes it follows slight trauma or local congestion due to coughing or sneezing but more usually it occurs spontaneously. Vascular diseases such as arteriosclerosis, hypertension and diabetes may be predisposing factors and it may also be seen in purpuric conditions. Such conditions should, of course, be excluded but in the vast majority of cases a subconjunctival haemorrhage is of no importance. The blood, which is usually in the interpalpebral portion of the conjunctiva as shown in 10.1, is gradually absorbed, changing colour from bright red to yellow. No local treatment is required.

Pingueculum

Exposure to wind and dust frequently causes degenerative changes in the interpalpebral conjunctiva, particularly in older people. The fibrous tissue undergoes hyaline degeneration and the elastic fibres proliferate to form a yellowish nodule, called a pingueculum, on the nasal side of the cornea, later appearing on the lateral side as well (10.2). It is avascular and is frequently unnoticed until an incidental conjunctivitis causes it to stand out clearly against the red background of dilated conjunctival vessels. A pingueculum causes no symptoms and requires no treatment.

Pterygium

Although a pterygium is primarily a corneal condition it is included here for comparison with pingueculum. Like the latter condition it is degenerative in nature and is found particularly in people who live in hot dusty climates. Pathologically a pterygium is a degeneration of Bowman's membrane and the superficial corneal lamellae together with replacement by vascularized tissue over which extends the conjunctival epithelium. The process begins at the nasal and temporal borders of the cornea and progresses towards the centre, taking with it a continuation of the conjunctival epithelium (10.3).

In the early stages a pterygium causes no symptoms but when it encroaches on the pupillary region vision is affected (10.4). If it is not treated serious visual disability will result.

Treatment consists in surgical removal and as recurrences are common many different procedures have been devised. Burying the apex beneath healthy conjunctiva is often effective in preventing recurrence.

Pemphigus

Pemphigus is one of a variety of mucocutaneous diseases of obscure aetiology in which blisters form in the skin and mucous membranes, including the conjunctiva. Ocular localization is particularly marked in the condition known as ocular pemphigoid or essential shrinkage of the conjunctiva. It is a relatively benign disease compared with the mortality of true pemphigus, but it is still a potentially blinding condition. The contraction of newly formed connective tissue under the conjunctiva results in bands of cicatricial tissue which in time obliterate the fornices of the conjunctiva, seal off the lacrimal ducts and lead to gross drying and keratinisation of the cornea.

Similar conjunctival and corneal changes ('cicatrising conjunctivitis') can be seen following other mucocutaneous disorders (e.g. erythema multiforme, graft-versus-host disease following organ transplantation), infections (e.g. trachoma), physical agents (e.g. alkali conjunctival burns) and drug reactions. 10.5 shows cicatricial bands in the conjunctiva and keratinisation on the ocular surface.

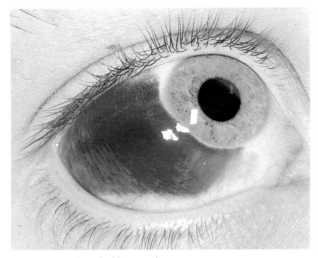

10.1 Subconjunctival haemorrhage

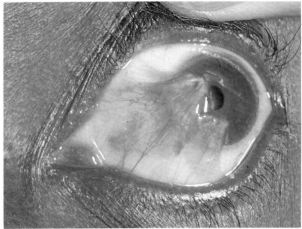

10.4 Pterygium (advanced)

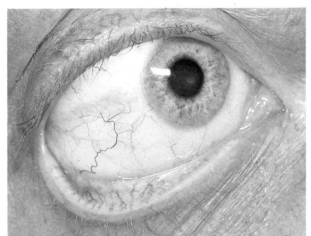

10.2 Pingueculum

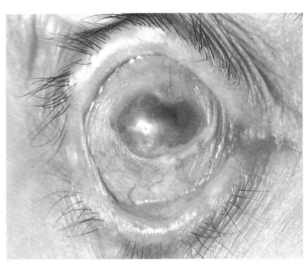

10.5 Ocular pemphigoid

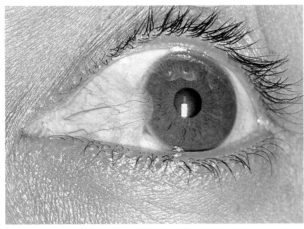

10.3 Pterygium (early)

Conjunctival and epibulbar tumours

The cornea being an avascular structure is very rarely the site of origin of a tumour. Many new growths however arise from the limbus (which is the site of transition from conjunctival to corneal epithelium) and these are grouped together under the title of epibulbar tumours.

Epithelial

Tumours of surface epithelium are unusual. They may be benign, precancerous or malignant. The latter include carcinoma in situ, squamous cell and muco-epidermoid. The carcinoma in situ occurs typically as an epibulbar tumour but may arise elsewhere in the conjunctiva or at the caruncle. At the limbus the tumour starts as a greyish nodule which extends over the cornea as a fleshy swelling demonstrated in 11.1. The corneal involvement causes a painful keratitis and frequently a secondary iridocyclitis. The tumour tends to grow fairly slowly and does not metastasise to the neighbouring lymph nodes until the later stages, so that the prognosis after enucleation is good.

Tumours and tumour-like lesions of the melanogenic system

Many different types of naevus exist including: junctional, compound, subepithelial, epitheloid and blue naevi. A cystic naevus is another type of benign epibulbar tumour which is really congenital in origin although it may not be apparent at birth. It grows very slowly unless malignant change supervenes. These tumours have derived from the end apparatus of sensory nerves and appear as yellowish plaques in the limbal region which on microscopical examination are found to consist of groups of large naevus cells in an alveolar formation. Golden granules of melanin are scattered throughout the tumour, being particularly abundant near the surface. 11.2 shows a typical cystic naevus — a yellowish ill-defined tumour with dilated conjunctival vessels supplying it. The cystic nature and frequent

granules can be clearly seen with the slit-lamp microscope. If the tumour is small and does not increase in size it can be left alone, but as the results of malignant change may be disastrous, complete excision should be considered.

Malignant melanoma

These may be epibulbar tumours or grow from any area of the conjunctiva arising in junctional, compound, blue naevi or primary acquired melanosis. Histologically they show the typical cellular structure of a malignant melanoma containing many blood vessels. The tumours are very malignant and tend to metastasise early, secondary deposits or orbital recurrences being common in spite of enucleation or even exenteration of the orbit. 11.3 shows an early tumour and 11.4 an advanced pedunculated tumour.

Vascular tumours

Telangiectasia, lymphangioma and haemangiomas occur in the conjunctiva. Haemangioma of the conjunctiva usually takes the form of the cavernous haemangioma consisting of spaces lined with endothelium containing blood and hyaline debris. The appearance of such a benign tumour is illustrated in 11.5. They may arise from conjunctival or from deeper episcleral vessels and can usually be excised satisfactorily.

Hamartomas and choristomas

Epibulbar dermoid — these tumours are present at birth and may be quite small initially, but slowly grow over the cornea. Histologically, they are covered by keratinized stratiform epithelium, often containing hair follicles, underneath which is a miscellaneous collection of elastic fibres, unstriated muscle, blood vessels and nerves. Such a growth is illustrated in 11.6. As they tend to increase in size they may cover the pupillary area and are best excised.

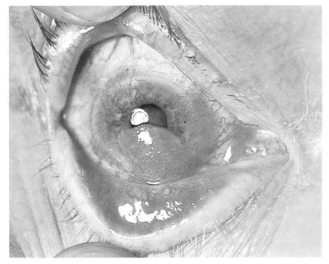

11.1 Epithelioma

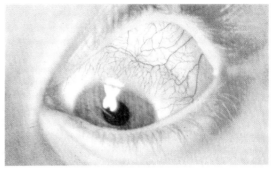

11.2 Cystic naevus of conjunctiva

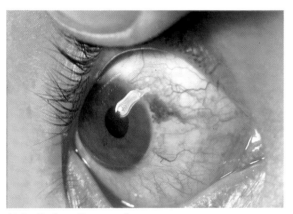

11.3 Early malignant melanoma

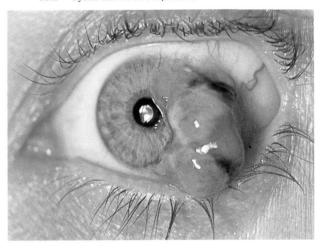

11.4 Advanced malignant melanoma

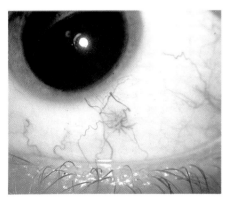

11.5 Haemangioma of conjunctiva

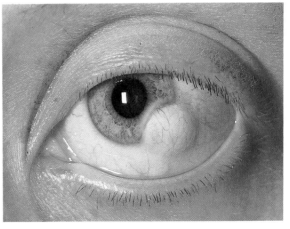

11.6 Epibulbar dermoid

12 The cornea: inflammations

Punctate epithelial keratitis

This is a common complication of some bacterial and viral infections. It may also follow trauma, contact lens wear, allergic conjunctivitis and keratoconjunctivitis sicca. The lesions are most easily recognized on slit-lamp examination after staining with fluorescein (12.1) or Rose Bengal. The commonest bacteria causing them is *Staphylococcus* in the form of sensitivity blepharo-keratoconjunctivitis. Common viruses implicated are adenovirus, tric, primary herpes simplex and varicella zoster. Symptoms are soreness and epiphora. Treatment is with the appropriate antiviral topically and when herpes simplex is excluded a dilute topical steroid.

Dendritic ulcer

This is a secondary manifestation of herpes simplex keratitis. Clinically the disease starts with an acutely painful eye, lacrimation and photophobia. The earliest corneal changes consist of fine epithelial opacities with a linear arrangement; these later turn into small vesicles which soon break down leaving raw areas which stain with fluorescein. The profile shows raised edges consisting of swollen and infected cells which stain with Rose Bengal. The pattern produced is of irregular branching lines with rounded tips. The corneal sensation is diminished and healing is slow without adequate treatment. 12.2 shows a branching pattern of an ulcer which has been stained with fluorescein and Rose Bengal. Treatment of choice is debridement followed by antiviral chemotherapy, such as IDU, Ara-A, trifluorothymidine, Acycloguanosine or Acyclovir. Steroid preparations have a very deleterious affect on the course of herpetic ulcers and should never be used unless the stroma is involved and even then should be combined with an antiviral.

Superficial stromal keratitis or nummular keratitis

This presents with blurring of vision and photophobia. It is characterized by areas of cellular infiltrate surrounded by haloes of stromal haze just beneath Bowman's membrane (12.3). It is caused by herpes zoster, late adenovirus and recurrent herpes simplex infections. The condition responds favourably to topical steroid (with herpes simplex antiviral cover when appropriate), but on suddenly stopping the therapy will relapse to produce denser opacities. Atypical organisms such as *Acanthamoebae* occasionally cause contact lens associated keratitis.

Interstitial keratitis

The active condition is rarely seen nowadays and in most cases the residual scarring is attributed to syphilis. It may be a manifestation of acquired syphilis, but is found most typically in young congenital syphilitics. It starts acutely with pain, lacrimation and photophobia; ciliary injection is marked and the cornea rapidly becomes hazy. Vessels now begin to grow into the cornea to produce the so-called salmon patch. The inflammation continues for 2–3 months then gradually subsides leaving a considerable degree of scarring (12.4). The vessels which have grown into the cornea never disappear and in time they cease to carry blood. Such ghost vessels can be seen on the slit-lamp and provide clear evidence of a previous interstitial keratitis.

Disciform keratitis

This is a marked infiltration and oedema of the central stroma (rarely it is eccentric) most frequently caused by herpes simplex virus but occasionally by herpes zoster. Symptoms are pronounced blurring of vision and photophobia. The epithelium appears hazy and rough with a disc shaped swelling extending posteriorly causing folds in Descemet's membrane and underlying depositions of keratitic precipitates (KP) (12.5). Treatment is with topical steroids and antiviral cover when appropriate.

Suppurative keratitis

This presents with severe pain and discharge from the eye. Biomicroscopically there is abscess formation in the corneal stroma usually with an overlying ulcer. It is caused by a bacterial secondary infection of a corneal ulcer such as may result from herpes simplex, incorrect contact lens wear or a neuroparalytic ulcer for nearly all eyes suffering from this condition have their health previously prejudiced in some way or another by previous disease. The corneal abscess may extend into a hypopyon where there is gross exudation of leucocytes and fibrin into the anterior chamber. 12.6 shows a typical hypopyon ulcer. Perforation of the cornea is always to be feared in these severe infections but fortunately Descemet's membrane is very resistant to invasion and intensive antibiotic therapy at an early stage is usually successful in averting such a catastrophe. Organisms commonly involved are *Streptococcus*, *Pneumococcus*, *Staphylococcus* and *Pseudomonas* (which tends to be the most severe).

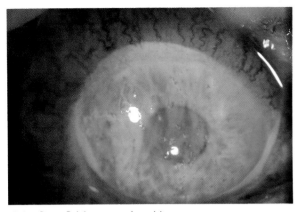

12.1 Superficial punctate keratitis

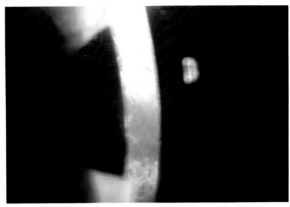

12.4 Interstitial keratitis

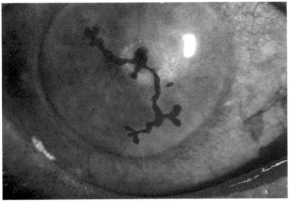

12.2 Dendritic ulcer

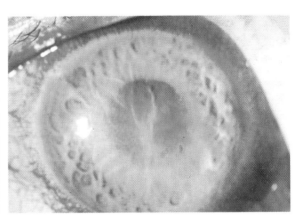

12.5 Disciform keratitis

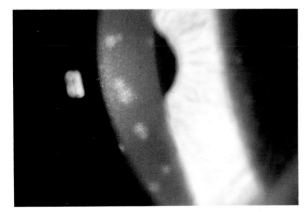

12.3 Adenovirus/stromal keratitis

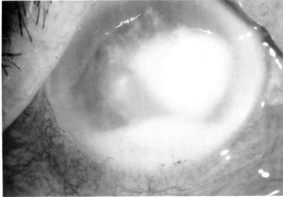

12.6 Hypopyon ulcer

13 The cornea: miscellaneous conditions

Keratoconus (conical cornea)

This very interesting condition has been included here as a degeneration of the cornea although its true aetiology is still uncertain. It may be developmental and some familial cases have been reported.

Typically the apical bulging of the cornea starts at puberty and increases slowly for several years. The only symptom is deterioration of vision due to the irregular myopic astigmatism caused by the changing corneal curvature. The shape of the cornea is best demonstrated by holding up the upper lid and asking the patient to look down so that the edge of the lower lid follows the corneal curvature across the midline. In the more severe cases the defect is obvious, as illustrated in 13.1 — a marked case of keratoconus with a normal eye for comparison. In the early stages the vision can be improved by spectacles but soon the refraction becomes too irregular for correction by ordinary lenses. This condition is one in which a most dramatic improvement in vision can be produced by contact lenses. It also responds well to corneal grafting.

Keratitis sicca

Deficiency of tear production leads to a characteristic picture in the cornea and conjunctiva. The conjunctiva loses its normal lustre and on microscopic examination with the slit-lamp the pre-corneal tear film can be seen to be reduced. Fine threads hang down from the corneal epithelium and there are ropy threads of mucus in the conjunctival sac. Staining with Rose Bengal shows up dry areas on the conjunctiva and punctate epithelial defects in the corneal epithelium (13.2). The condition is most commonly associated with Sjögren's syndrome and affects middle-aged women. The lacrimal glands, salivary glands and joints are involved. The aetiology is unknown, but an auto-immune mechanism may be responsible.

There is no cure for the chronic tear deficiency in severe keratitis sicca. Artificial tear lubricants offer partial symptomatic relief. Deliberate surgical closure of the lacrimal puncta may help moisten the eyes by preventing tear drainage. Treatable local factors exacerbating ocular irritation should be removed (such as blepharitis, trichiasis etc.).

Band opacity

Calcium salts can be deposited in any site of long-standing hyaline degeneration but are most commonly seen in the cornea following a 'band-shaped degeneration'. In this condition a band of hyaline degeneration stretches across the cornea in the interpalpebral region. Such a case in which calcareous change has developed is illustrated in 13.3. Some cases of band keratopathy are due to hypercalcaemia. Most cases of band keratopathy follow ocular diseases such as uveitis and phthisis, and are not caused by hypercalcaemia.

Dystrophies

These rare conditions have been described under many different names but can be divided roughly into those affecting primarily the endothelium and epithelium and those affecting the corneal stroma.

It is not uncommon to find some bedewing of the endothelium in elderly patients but this rarely causes any interference with vision. Fuchs' dystrophy, which is illustrated in 13.4, starts with a similar endothelial change but progresses to involve the epithelium as well, causing marked oedema and deterioration of vision. The central hazy oedematous area is well shown in 13.5.

Many of the stromal dystrophies are familial, the first signs appearing at puberty and slowly progressing throughout life. They are characterized by scattered hyaline changes in the anterior layers of the cornea and the patches may be arranged in many different patterns, lattice-like white lines, rosettes, white rings and other variations.

13.6 is a photograph of a case of Groenouw's corneal dystrophy which has been chosen to illustrate this group of diseases. Whitish spots which may have a ring shape are scattered over the central area of the cornea beneath Bowman's membrane. It is a familial condition and progresses slowly. Corneal grafting offers good hope of visual improvement.

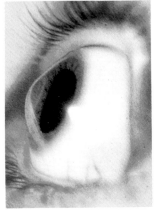
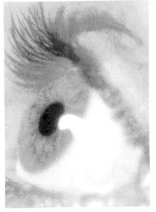

13.1 Keratoconus

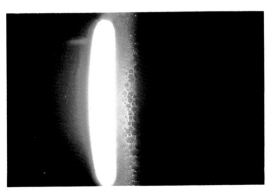

13.4 Fuchs' dystrophy

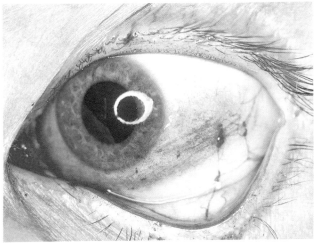

13.2 Keratitis sicca

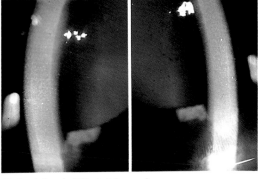

13.5 Advanced Fuchs' dystrophy

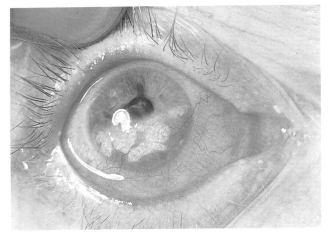

13.3 Calcareous degeneration

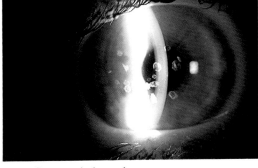

13.6 Groenouw's dystrophy

14 *The sclera*

Blue sclerotics

Congenital thinning of the sclera, allowing the underlying pigment epithelium to show through and thus give a blue colour, is associated with fragilitas ossium and otosclerosis.

Episcleritis

The episclera is a fibro-elastic structure, the vascular coat on the surface of the sclera providing for part of its nutrition. Inflammation here takes two forms: the commoner, simple episcleritis and nodular episcleritis. Thirty per cent are associated with general medical conditions such as collagen disease, herpes zoster, gout and syphilis.

Simple episcleritis is characterized by a very acute onset and is usually mild in course, sectoral, recurrent and resolves rapidly (14.1).

Nodular episcleritis is a localized raised mobile area of inflammation usually near the limbus (14.2). The nodules may be single or multiple and the condition is usually recurrent. Topical steroids will speed up the process of resolution in both conditions.

Scleritis

The sclera consists of collagen and much elastic tissue, therefore it suffers from chronic granulomatous and destructive lesions which affect collagen. Scleritis is manifested clinically by severe pain and destruction of tissues, even leading to loss of the eye. The overlying episclera is always involved. It may be classified anatomically into anterior and posterior, and again into diffuse, nodular or necrotizing. Diffuse and nodular scleritis are characterized by severe pain and a bluish red area of inflammation in the deeper layers of the sclera (14.3). They are commonest in the 4–5th decades and in women more than men. They are bilateral in 50 per cent of cases: 21 per cent are associated with rheumatoid arthritis and other collagen diseases; 12 per cent with ankylosing spondylitis; and 15 per cent with herpes zoster, TB, syphilis, gout and Reiter's disease.

Necrotizing scleritis occurs in two forms — one of which shows severe inflammation and pain, and the other, scleromalacia perforans, has practically no painful or inflammatory component (14.4). Forty per cent are associated with severe polyarticular rheumatoid arthritis. Complications of all types of scleritis include keratitis, uveitis, glaucoma, cataract and exudative retinal detachment. Scleral thinning and necrosis occur in nearly all cases.

Topical steroids may help but are usually insufficient alone. Systemic nonsteroid anti-inflammatory agents are usually employed such as oxyphenbutazone and indomethacin. They are employed to suppress the destructive processes until a natural remission occurs in the disease. If these treatments fail systemic steroids are necessary and prednisolone is especially effective.

Staphyloma

The normal adult sclera is able to resist stretching by a raised intra-ocular pressure, but if the sclera is weakened by impairment of nutrition or by inflammation it may stretch and thin, usually in the region of the ciliary body (14.5).

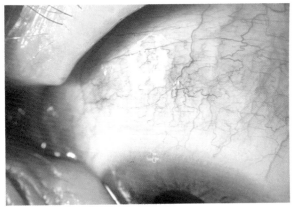

14.1 Simple episcleritis

14.2 Nodular episcleritis

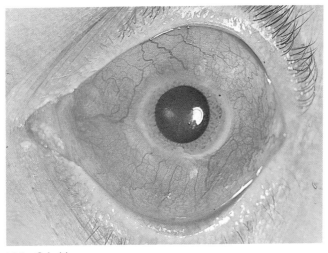

14.3 Scleritis

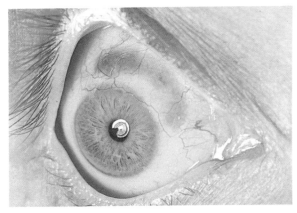

14.4 Scleromalacia perforans

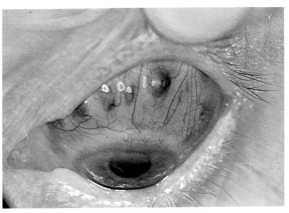

14.5 Staphyloma

15 *The iris and ciliary body: inflammations*

Although many causes are known for anterior uveitis, the aetiology is still obscure in many cases and a simple clinical classification into acute and chronic is as useful as any.

Acute iridocyclitis

Pain, photophobia, lacrimation and blurring of vision are the classical symptoms of an acute iridocyclitis. The eye is red, the injection being ciliary in type with a deep flush all round the limbus (15.1). The engorgement of vessels frequently involves those of the iris and, as always in an acute inflammatory process, the hyperaemia is followed by an exudation of protein and cells, in this case into the aqueous of the anterior chamber. The oedema and vascularity of the iris cause a blurring of the iris pattern and the normal coloration becomes less clear. The aqueous humour in a quiet eye is optically empty, which means that if a bright beam of light is thrown across the anterior chamber the aqueous appears dark. When exudate is present, however, some light is reflected back from the protein and cellular elements, giving rise to the so-called 'aqueous flare', in the same way that dust in the air shows in shafts of sunlight. Cells can be seen floating in the beam. Clumps of exudate and cells settle on the posterior surface of the cornea as keratic precipitates — a sure sign of cyclitis, but one which it usually requires a loupe or microscope to detect (15.5).

Inflammatory irritation of the pupil causes it to constrict, and in the later stages it may become adherent to the anterior surface of the lens (posterior synechiae). Under the influence of a mydriatic the pupil dilates, but when it is partially adherent an irregular shape results, as is seen in 15.2.

The commonest aetiological association with acute anterior uveitis is ankylosing spondylitis or the chronic stage of Reiter's disease. Both conditions are much more common in men than in women and in both a chronic urogenital infection probably precedes the typical changes in the sacro-iliac joints and lumbar spine (15.3). In Reiter's disease the metatarsophalangeal joints may also be affected. The cause of this association between urogenital disease, arthritis and uveitis is not known, but it may be a virus infection, perhaps associated with a hypersensitivity type of immunological reaction.

Other cases may follow upper respiratory disease of viral origin such as influenza, but in a large proportion of cases (particularly in women) no cause is found.

Sarcoidosis is sometimes accompanied by an acute anterior uveitis, particularly in young adults with hilar adenopathy.

A rare but distinctive type of uveitis is seen as part of the symptom complex known as Behçet's disease. Typically the patient presents with an acute anterior uveitis, with hypopyon, in one eye (15.4). Sooner or later the disease recurs and affects both eyes, leading eventually to blindness. Although it is difficult to see the fundus, a retinitis or retinal vasculitis is usually present. Recurrent ulceration of the mucous membranes of the mouth and/or genitalia is a typical feature, but other systems — the skin, the joints and the central nervous system, for example — are often involved. The disease seems to be more common in the Middle East and is probably viral in origin. Systemic steroid therapy helps to control the recurrent inflammation but no curative treatment is known.

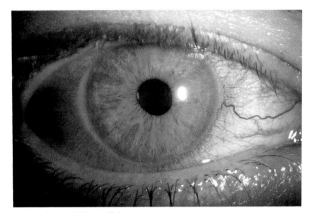

15.1 Acute iridocyclitis

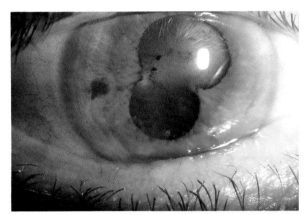

15.2 Posterior synechiae

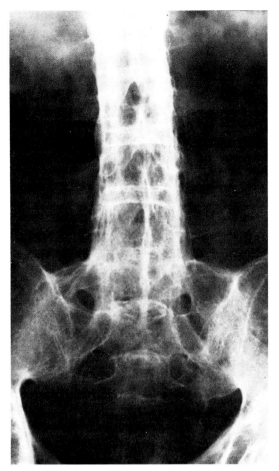

15.3 Ankylosing spondylitis

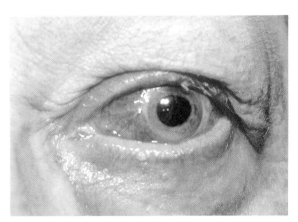

15.4 Hypopyon uveitis

15 The iris and ciliary body: inflammations (cont.)

Chronic anterior uveitis

Two main types occur: one, caused by granulomatous diseases such as tuberculosis and sarcoidosis, is characterized by severe destructive lesions, often with nodules in the iris, numerous posterior synechiae and large 'mutton-fat' keratic precipitates (15.5 and 15.6). The other type of chronic anterior uveitis is a quiet process involving more particularly the ciliary body: a chronic cyclitis. The most important clinical entity in this group is the condition known as heterochromic uveitis.

In the granulomatous type of chronic anterior uveitis, sarcoidosis is the commonest aetiological factor in England. Tuberculosis, brucellosis, leptospirosis, syphilis and such conditions as onchocerciasis may be more common in countries with a higher incidence of these diseases. In sarcoidosis multiple nodules in the iris, and granulomas extending into the angle of the anterior chamber, give a characteristic appearance; skin lesions are common (15.7) and hilar gland enlargement with or without infiltration of the lung fields is diagnostic (15.8). The salivary and lacrimal glands may also be affected.

Heterochromic uveitis

Heterochromic uveitis is an interesting condition of unknown aetiology, with characteristic (though often unrecognized) clinical features. Typically the patient is a young adult who complains of slight mistiness of vision and floating spots in one eye. The heterochromia may be very slight in early cases, particularly when the normal colour of the iris is grey or blue. Usually the affected eye is lighter in colour (15.9), but when the stromal atrophy, the cause of the change in colour, is extreme the affected eye may appear darker because the pigment epithelium is more exposed. Translucent, non-pigmented keratic precipitates can be seen on the slit-lamp and there are usually some fine particles or cells in the aqueous. The iris shows stromal atrophy and on transillumination through the pupil the pigment epithelium has a moth-eaten appearance at the pupillary margin. On gonioscopy fine vessels can be seen in the trabecular region. Anterior vitreous opacities are always present. Posterior cortical lens changes are always seen and may eventually progress to complete opacity of the lens (15 .9). Secondary glaucoma develops in some cases.

Slight ptosis and enophthalmos are not uncommon on the affected side (15.10), and a lesion of the sympathetic supply has been postulated in such cases, perhaps as part of the wider syndrome of status dysraphicus. Anti-inflammatory treatment with steroids has no appreciable effect, supporting the view that heterochromic uveitis is a dystrophic condition rather than an inflammation.

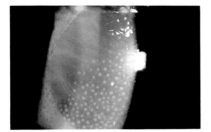

15.5 Keratic precipitates

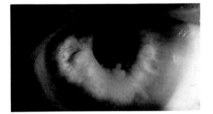

15.6 Iris nodules due to sarcoidosis

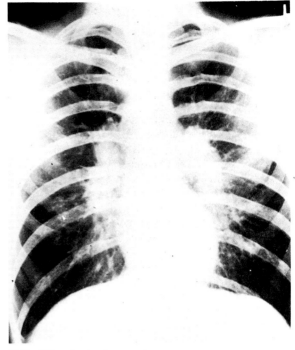

15.8 Hilar gland enlargement

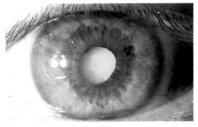

15.9 Iris stromal atrophy and mature cataract

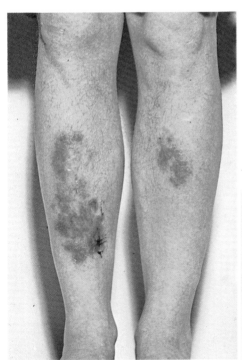

15.7 Erythema nodosum skin lesions in systemic sarcoidosis

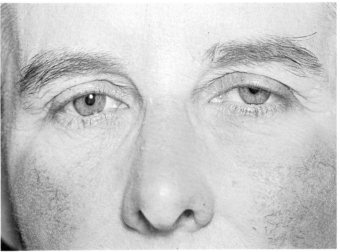

15.10 Heterochromic uveitis

16 *The iris and ciliary body: neoplasms*

The lens, being an avascular structure is never the site of a new growth but the iris and ciliary body may be the site of tumours similar to those occurring in the choroid, the commonest being neuro-ectodermal in origin.

Naevus or benign melanoma

Pigment flecks or freckles on the iris are very common and are usually of no importance. The larger naevi as illustrated in 16.1 may, however, grow and undergo malignant change. Naevi of the ciliary body cannot be seen clinically but may be observed histologically in eyes sectioned for other reasons.

Leiomyoma of the iris

This is a rather controversial lesion from the histological viewpoint and is characterized by closely packed bundles of long spindle-shaped cells resembling a melanoma but arising from the muscle of the iris. Clinically it is impossible to distinguish from a melanoma. It is a lightly pigmented yellowish tumour which grows slowly and is relatively benign. 16.2 is a photograph of such a tumour accompanied by its angiogram. Metastases do not occur but the neoplasm may recur locally if not completely removed or may bleed causing a hyphaema.

Malignant melanoma of the ciliary body

This is usually unnoticed until it extends forward as a pigmented mass at the base of the iris or unless lens changes occur causing visual deterioration. The tumour can usually be seen through the fully dilated pupil. Malignant melanomas of the ciliary body tend to infiltrate the sclera and may be seen emerging under the conjunctiva at the limbus. 16.3 shows a malignant melanoma which has extended forward over the base of the iris and outwards through the sclera.

Malignant melanoma of the iris

This is a rare disease and the majority of those reported have arisen from a pre-existing naevus. The latter may appear unchanged for many years and then quite suddenly increase its size and become more vascular (16.4). There are several morphological types. 16.5 shows a sclerosing type where there is distortion of the pupil. Advanced growth spreads into the ciliary body and tends to block the angle of the anterior chamber causing glaucoma. In the early stages it may be possible to excise the sector of iris containing the tumour but later on it is necessary to enucleate the eye.

Metastatic tumours of the iris

Iris metastases are uncommon. They usually arise from primary tumours of the breast or bronchus.

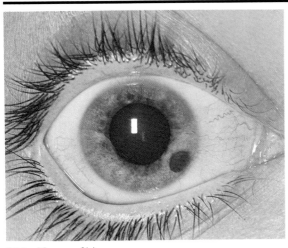

16.1 Naevus of iris

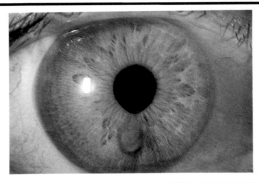

A

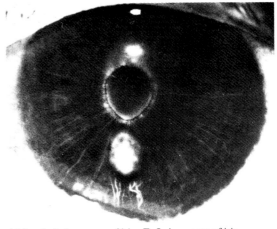

B

16.2 **A** Leiomyoma of iris. **B** Leiomyoma of iris (fluorescein)

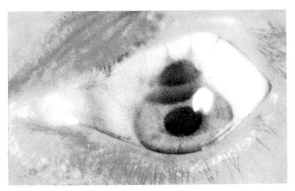

16.3 Infiltrating melanoma of choroid

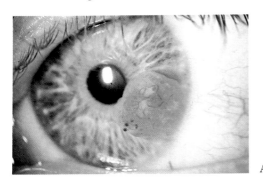

A

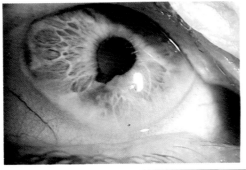

B

16.4 **A** Vascular malignant melanoma of iris. **B** Vascular malignant melanoma of iris (fluorescein)

16.5 Sclerosing malignant melanoma of iris

17 *Trauma to the anterior segment*

Perforating wounds

Perforating wounds of the cornea frequently involve the iris and lens. The pupil constricts in response to injury, and as the aqueous leaks out of the corneal wound the iris tends to prolapse through the opening. If the wound is small, the prolapse acts as a plug and allows the anterior chamber to reform. Such an injury is illustrated in 17.1, in which the knuckle of prolapsed iris shows as a dark blob at the site of perforation of the cornea — in this case near the limbus at seven o'clock. If the patient is seen within a few hours and the nature of the perforating object is such that infection is unlikely, it is advisable to replace the prolapse and suture the corneal wound.

Iridodialysis

The thinnest part of the iris is at its origin from the ciliary body, and a contusion of the eye may tear the iris at this point, causing an iridodialysis. Such an injury is illustrated in 17.2, in which the iris can be seen detached from the ciliary body in an arc over the lower segment. The pupil is flattened in the region of the dialysis.

Hyphaema

Blood may enter the anterior chamber following injuries (hyphaema) (17.3). The management of hyphaema is controversial, but may include bed rest, eyepatching, topical steroids, cycloplegia and, in severe cases, surgical clot evacuation. Secondary glaucoma and permanent corneal blood staining may follow hyphaema.

Dislocation of the lens

Contusion injuries may rupture the zonule of the lens and cause its dislocation. Usually the lens is displaced laterally or downwards, as in 17.4, where the edge of the opaque cataractous lens shows clearly in the pupillary area. This illustration also shows a hypertrophy of black iris pigment over the front surface of the iris. More rarely the lens is dislocated forwards into the anterior chamber, where it is very liable to block the drainage of aqueous and cause a secondary glaucoma.

Foreign bodies in the eye

A wide variety of foreign bodies may enter the eye in injuries. The commonest are small fragments of metal from hammer-and-chisel accidents or from moving parts of machinery. It must be emphasized that the immediate symptoms of this type of injury may be slight, and a small corneal wound is easily overlooked. Radiographs of the eye should be taken after every injury in which it is at all possible that a foreign body may have entered the eye, as any small fragment which has perforated the globe will almost certainly be metallic. Glass may not be revealed by radiography, but usually the history will suggest the possibility of its presence, and examination with a slit-lamp microscope may enable it to be seen in the anterior segment.

17.5 is an illustration of a small metallic foreign body which has entered the anterior chamber through the cornea.

Siderosis bulbi

If an iron-containing foreign body is retained within the eye, the iron is slowly liberated, causing dark brown pigmentation of the iris, cornea and lens (17.6). Atrophic changes occur in the uveal tract and retina and lens opacities may progress to a mature cataract.

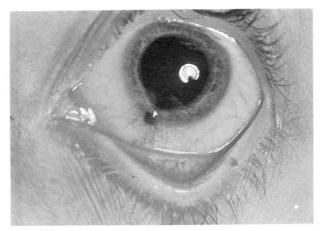

17.1 Perforating wound, prolapsed iris

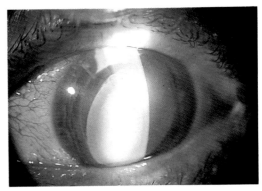

17.4 Disclocation of lens

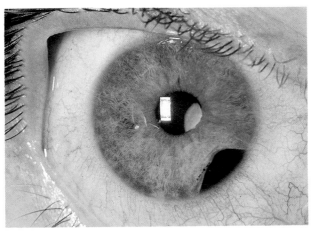

17.2 Iridodialysis and sectorial cataract

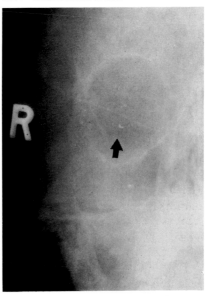

17.5 X-ray intra-ocular foreign body

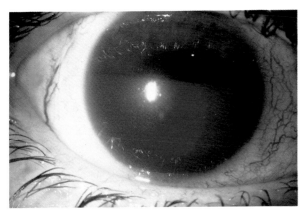

17.3 Hyphaema

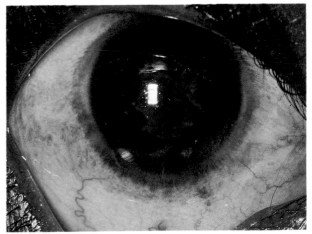

17.6 Siderosis bulbi

18 *The lens*

Congenital cataract

It will be remembered that the lens is ectodermal in origin and that new fibres are formed by the elongation of the epithelial cells at the equator. Thus, as more lens fibres are laid down, the earlier fibres become centrally placed. Any injury or disturbance of metabolism may render opaque the fibres which are being formed at that time, and therefore the position of the opacity in the lens gives an accurate date to the incident. New fibres continue to be formed throughout life, but very much more slowly than in the foetus.

Congenital lens opacities of many varieties have been recognized and described since the early days of ophthalmology, but remained pathological curiosities until the work of Gregg threw new light on their aetiology and, indeed, that of many other congenital defects. In 1941, Gregg noticed that following an epidemic of rubella many of the children whose mothers had contracted the disease in the first two months of pregnancy were born with cataract, sometimes associated with congenital heart disease.

Unless the lens is completely opaque congenital cataracts may not be noticed until the child is found to have a visual defect.

18.1 illustrates a zonular cataract, one of the many types of congenital lens change. Some of the fibres laid down during development are abnormal and form a partially opaque zone between the embryonic nucleus and the cortex of the lens. Such congenital cataracts are usually bilateral and surgical treatment is indicated if the reduction in visual acuity is sufficient to hinder normal development.

Small punctate bluish opacities are a common finding in normal eyes, and represent occasional lens fibres which have not developed normally. If such opacities are marked, they are known as blue-dot cataracts (18.2). Vision is rarely affected.

Neonatal cataract is frequently seen in galactosaemia, which is a serious and treatable disorder.

Coronary cataract

Coronary cataract is a type of development cataract appearing soon after puberty. Numerous club-shaped whitish opacities can be seen in the peripheral cortex of the lens, often associated with blue-dot changes (18.3). Such appearances can be found in many people, but as they are peripheral and of very slow progression they rarely produce any visual defect.

Ectopia lentis

If the suspensory ligament of the lens is absent, the whole lens becomes displaced away from the weak portion. Such displacement is called ectopia lentis and occurs not uncommonly as a congenital and often hereditary defect (18.4). When the pupil is well dilated, it is possible to see the fundus ophthalmoscopically through the lens and also round the edge of the lens.

Ectopia lentis may be a component of a widespread mesodermal defect known as Marfan's syndrome, characterized by an elongation of the long bones, particularly of the hands and feet, undeveloped musculature and infantilism. The long, spidery fingers have given the disease the name of arachnodactyly. 18.5 is a photograph of the hands of a six-year-old boy with this condition. The ectopia is often associated with myopia and astigmatism, and the weakened zonule predisposes to traumatic dislocation of the lens.

Persistent hyaloid artery

Some remnants of the hyaloid artery can be seen on the posterior surface of the lens in a high proportion of normal people, but occasionally a complete tract can be made out running from the posterior surface of the lens to the optic disc (18.6).

Senile cataract

Some degree of lenticular sclerosis is always present in old age and can be recognized by the increased scattering of light from the lens. This is evidenced by the slightly greyish appearance of the pupil in old people compared with the jet black pupil of young people. The effect on vision, however, is insignificant, and usually no opacity will be seen with the ophthalmoscope.

Senile cataract usually commences in the peripheral cortical areas and can be seen with a +12 D lens in the ophthalmoscope as dark spokes at the periphery of the lens against the red reflex from the fundus. 18.7 is

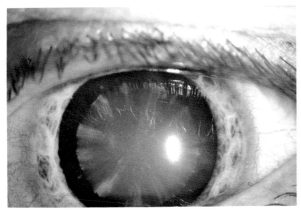

18.1 Zonular cataract

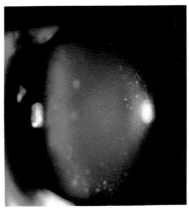

18.2 Blue dot cataract

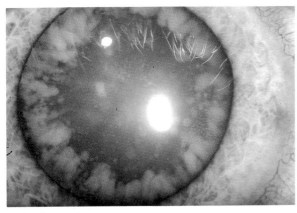

18.3 Coronary cataract

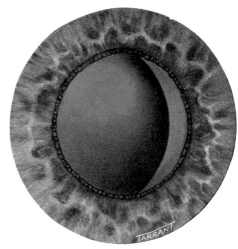

18.4 Ectopia lentis

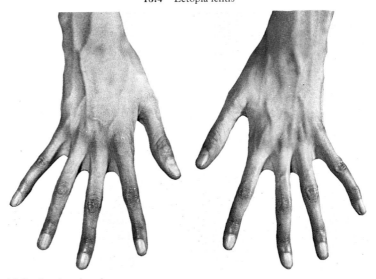

18.5 Arachnodactyly

a photograph of a typical senile cataract in which the peripheral spokes and opacities are silhouetted against reflected light from the fundus. Nuclear sclerosis will produce much more serious interference with vision and will require operative treatment earlier than the more usual peripheral opacities.

With modern operative technique it is no longer necessary to wait for a cataract to become 'ripe' (i.e. for complete opacification of the lens) before it can be extracted, and the criterion for operation now is the visual disability of the patient.

Diabetic cataract

Although it is common to find senile lens changes at an earlier age in diabetics than in other patients, a true diabetic cataract is rare. When it does occur, it is usually in a young person and often progresses very rapidly, the lens becoming completely opaque in a matter of weeks. The opacity is in the superficial layers of the cortex and consists of numerous white spots and fluid vacuoles, as shown in 18.8.

Complicated cataract

Any severe disease of the inner eye, such as a long-standing uveitis, detached retina or intra-ocular neoplasm, may derange the metabolic processes of the lens sufficiently to cause cataract. Chronic uveitis is the most common offender; 18.9 shows an eye with uveitis and a mature cataract. The upper part of the iris has been removed surgically, but elsewhere it has an atrophic appearance and is adherent to the lens by numerous posterior synechiae. The changes start at the posterior pole and often show a typical polychromatic lustre when seen with the slit-lamp microscope. 18.10 shows posterior cortical changes in the lens complicating a uveitis, as seen by slit illumination.

Drug induced cataract

Posterior polar changes similar to those seen in complicated cataract may result from prolonged treatment with corticosteroid drugs either given systemically or locally as drops. Phenothiazine compounds may be deposited on the anterior surface of the lens but fortunately have little if any effect on vision.

Cataract surgery

Cataract surgery is usually performed on patients in whom lenticular opacities cause significant visual impairment. A small number of patients have cataract surgery for lens induced glaucoma or uveitis, or where the lens prevents the ophthalmologist from treating retinal disorders. It is important to diagnose or exclude diabetes mellitus in patients with cataract.

Cataract surgery can be performed under general or local anaesthesia as an inpatient or outpatient procedure. There are several methods of removing the lenticular opacity and treating the resultant reduction of overall focussing power of the eye. The lens has a solid nucleus (which increases in size with age), a semi-solid cortex around the nucleus, and a thin capsule.

Mydriatic drops are instilled preoperatively. In all cases the surgeon makes an incision in the peripheral cornea or anterior sclera. The entire lens may be removed in one piece including its capsule (intracapsular surgery) or the lens may be removed through a hole in the capsule leaving most of the capsule intact (extracapsular surgery) (18.11). All modern cataract surgery is performed using a binocular operating microscope, and most are performed using the extracapsular technique.

An incision of $10^{1}/_{2}$ mm or so long is required to deliver the lens nucleus in intracapsular or conventional extracapsular surgery. A much smaller incision can be used if the entire lens is liquid enough to aspirate, as is the case in youth, or if the lens is cut up with a suction cutter or fragmented with a specialised ultrasonic probe (18.12). Soft cortex remnants are aspirated, taking care to preserve the posterior part of the lens capsule in extracapsular surgery (18.13).

An artificial intraocular lens can be implanted at this stage. These lenses are normally supported by the original lens capsule (18.14). Alternative intraocular implant designs can be clipped to the iris, or supported by the angle between the iris and cornea.

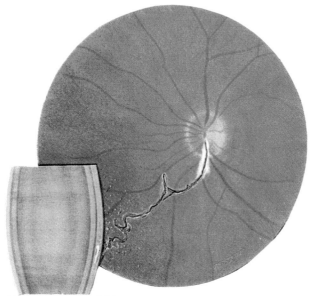

18.6   Persistent hyaloid artery

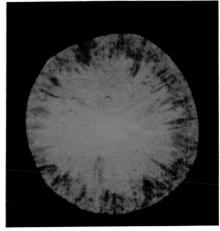

18.7   Senile cataract

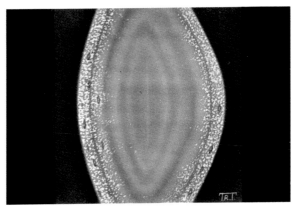

18.8   Diabetic cataract

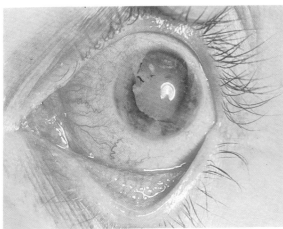

18.9   Secondary cataract due to uveitis

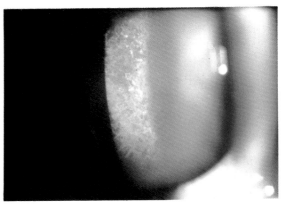

18.10   Post cortical lens opacities

These alternative designs are useful where the posterior capsule is incomplete or absent following removal of a cataract.

The wound is sutured, and the patient commenced on topical antibiotic and steroid drops. It is important that the patient does not rub or injure the eye whilst the wound is healing. Optical correction is usually prescribed approximately 2 months after surgery, though the timing may vary depending on the surgical technique used. Patients who have not had an intra-ocular lens implant frequently achieve a better optical correction with a contact lens than with spectacles.

Postoperative discomfort

Most patients experience little or no discomfort following surgery. A mild anterior uveitis is usual and is treated with topical steroid drops with or without a mydriatic. Infective endophthalmitis is an uncommon complication after cataract surgery. The patient experiences considerable pain, blurring and lid swelling within days of surgery. There is an intense uveitis with leakage of cells and fibrin into the anterior chamber, frequently with hypopyon formation (18.15). Painful corneal oedema may follow cataract surgery and this may benefit from corneal grafting if it persists.

The wound and sutures cause a transient minor foreign body sensation. The wound is usually reasonably secure after about six weeks. Nylon sutures tend to degrade slowly, and may snap many months after surgery. Sutures are removed if their snapped ends are protruding and causing discomfort.

Postoperative blurring

Some patients experience optical blurring until spectacle correction is ordered. Approximately 25% of patients develop slowly progressive thickening of the posterior lens capsule following cataract surgery and this opacification may be treated by laser capsulotomy. Corneal oedema, anterior uveitis, macular oedema and retinal detachment may also cause a drop in vision following cataract surgery.

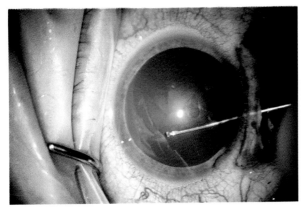

18.11 Anterior capsulotomy

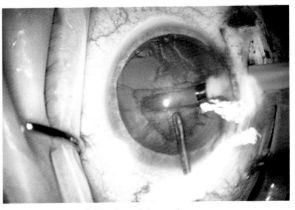

18.12 Phacoemulsification of the nucleus

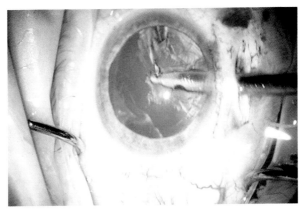

18.13 Aspiration of cortex

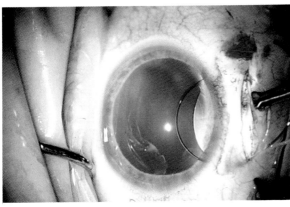

18.14 Intraocular lens implantation

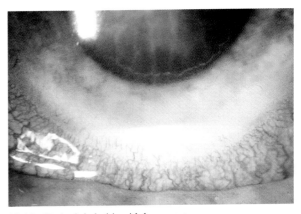

18.15 Endophthalmitis with hypopyon

19 *Glaucoma*

The normal ocular tension

The intraocular pressure can be estimated by the use of a tonometer, which measures the tension in the ocular coats.

There is no one figure which expresses the upper limit of normal for all eyes. As in all biological measurements, normal values are spread over a considerable range, and tonometric surveys on normal populations have shown that ocular tension is no exception (19.1). The actual values from different surveys vary slightly, depending on the methods used, but the distribution of tensions approximates to a Gaussian curve with a mean between 15 and 16 mm Hg and a standard deviation of about ±2.5. A distribution of this type means that the probability of any particular ocular tension can be assessed in terms of its distance from the mean value. The values for 95% of the population will lie between plus and minus two standard deviations from the mean. Over 99% will be covered by three standard deviations from the mean. Ocular tensions of over 21 mm Hg are therefore likely to be found in about 2.5% of a normal population. A tension above 24 mm Hg is only likely to be found in about one in 200 of a normal population, and the probability that tensions above this level are normal decreases as the tension becomes higher. The ocular tension varies with age, sex and time of day and too much significance should not be attached to a single reading.

Glaucoma

Glaucoma is a condition in which raised intraocular pressure causes pathological changes in the eye. It may be caused by a recognized ocular lesion such as a neoplasm or inflammation, in which case it is called *secondary glaucoma*. A typical example is shown in 19.2. Posterior synechiae have sealed the pupillary opening to the anterior surface of the lens, causing an increase in pressure in the posterior chamber which bulges the iris forward (iris bombé) so that the periphery of the iris closes the angle of the anterior chamber, effectively blocking the exit of the aqueous humour and causing secondary glaucoma.

Primary glaucoma, in which the exciting cause is less obvious, can be divided into three main types: congenital glaucoma, chronic simple glaucoma and closed angle glaucoma.

Congenital glaucoma

In this condition there is a failure of normal development of the tissues at the angle of the anterior chamber which impedes the outflow of aqueous humour from the eye. It is more common in boys than girls and is usually apparent during the first year of life. At this age the outer coats of the eye are soft and expand under the influence of the raised pressure, giving a large eye with an increase in corneal diameter (19.3) — thus the name 'buphthalmos'. This may be enough to call attention to the abnormality, but usually the baby shuns the light and corneal oedema disturbs the bright lustre of the normal cornea, producing a 'ground-glass' appearance. In a baby a corneal diameter of 12 mm or more, corneal oedema and raised tension are diagnostic features. Medical treatment is of little value, but the operation of goniotomy, in which an incision is made into the tissue of the angle, is often successful in restoring outflow. The appearance of the abnormal angle is shown in 19.4.

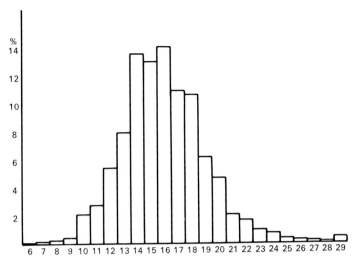

19.1 Frequency distribution of ocular tensions

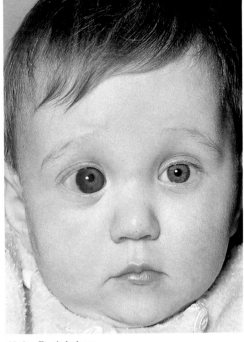

19.3 Buphthalmos

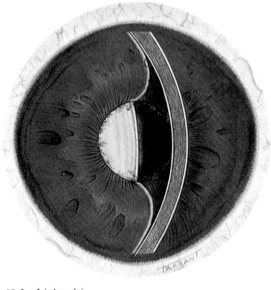

19.2 Iris bombé

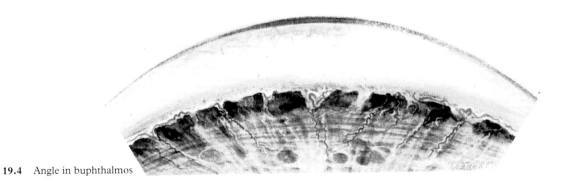

19.4 Angle in buphthalmos

Glaucoma (cont.)

Investigation of glaucoma

The first decision to be made in the investigation of a case of suspected glaucoma is whether the angle is open or closed or so narrow that closure is likely. The angle is hidden from direct observation by the overlapping of the sclera at the limbus. If, however, the refraction of the cornea is cancelled by the application of a suitable contact lens, it is possible to view the angle microscopically. The contact lens may be dome-shaped, as in the Koeppe and Barkan designs, or conical, as in the Goldmann type, the optical principles of which are illustrated in 19.5. The dome-shaped lenses are designed for use with a hand-held binocular loupe or microscope, while the Goldmann lens is for use with the slit-lamp microscope.

In an open angle the end of Descemet's membrane in the cornea appears as a pale line marking the anterior insertion of the trabeculae (19.6). Blood may show in the canal of Schlemm as a pink band beneath the trabeculae, and if the angle is wide the root of the ciliary body can be seen. In a narrow angle only Schwalbe's line and a glimpse of the trabeculae are visible (19.7).

If the angle is wide, the diagnosis of chronic simple glaucoma will depend on tonometry, the appearance of the optic disc, and visual field studies, which must include a careful examination of the central field. The typical cupping of the disc in chronic simple glaucoma is shown in 19.8.

In cases with a narrow angle the diagnosis depends on the demonstration of a raised tension with irido-corneal contact or a history of typical symptoms and the ability to provoke a mild attack under controlled conditions by a test such as the dark-room test.

Chronic simple glaucoma

Chronic simple glaucoma is a condition in which there is a slow increase in resistance to outflow of the aqueous humour, causing a chronic rise in intraocular pressure which embarrasses the blood supply to the optic nerve with resulting atrophy of nerve fibres and cupping of the optic disc (19.8).

There is strong evidence for a genetic abnormality, but the expression of the defect is usually delayed until later life. Both sexes are affected, men slightly more often than women, and the incidence rises sharply after the age of 60. Symptoms are slight or absent in the early stages; the chronic rise in pressure does not cause pain, and the initial field defects do not affect central vision and often remain unrecognized until a large amount of field has been lost. As treatment can only prevent further loss, early diagnosis is of great importance, and tonometry should be part of the routine examination of all patients over the age of 40.

The earliest evidence of visual field defects is usually found in the so-called arcuate area about 10 degrees above or below fixation which corresponds to the distribution of optic nerve fibres (19.9A). Arcuate scotomas above and below the horizontal often do not coincide at the 180 degree meridian and the result is a step in the defect nasally. The scotomas extend peripherally and if the disease progresses unchecked the patient may be left with only a small central visual field (19.9B).

The management of chronic simple glaucoma is aimed at reducing the intraocular pressure to arrest or slow the decline in visual loss. Topical pilocarpine, beta adrenoreceptor blockers and adrenergic agonists may be used as well as oral carbonic anhydrase inhibitors.

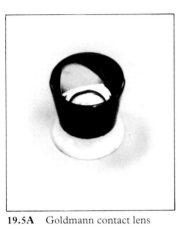

19.5A Goldmann contact lens

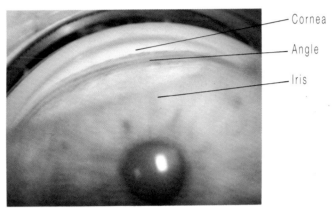

Cornea

Angle

Iris

19.6 Normal broad angle

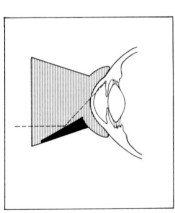

19.5B Optical principle

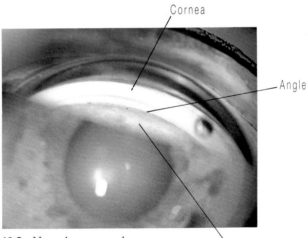

Cornea

Angle

Iris

19.7 Normal narrow angle

Surgery is usually reserved for cases where medical therapy fails to control glaucoma, or where the treatment required to control glaucoma is associated with unacceptable drug-induced side effects.

Trabeculectomy is the commonest surgical procedure used to treat open angle glaucoma. This procedure involves forming a new channel for aqueous through a partial thickness hole in the sclera from the anterior chamber into the subconjunctival space. Newer modifications of this technique involve the use of antimetabolites locally to prevent scarring along the new aqueous path, and the use of prosthetic tubes to bypass scar tissue.

Closed-angle glaucoma

This type of glaucoma occurs in eyes which have an anatomical predisposition by reason of a shallow anterior chamber and a narrow angle between the base of the iris and the peripheral cornea. As the lens grows with age the iris is pushed further forwards to such a degree that the resistance to flow of aqueous through the pupil is enough to cause an increase in pressure behind the iris, causing the weaker periphery of the iris to bulge forward until it comes into contact with

the trabecular region and seals off the exit of aqueous. A rapid rise in intraocular pressure follows, causing pain and blurring of vision from corneal oedema which produces by diffraction the appearance of rainbow haloes round small sources of light. If the angle remains closed the blood supply to the optic nerve is seriously impeded and vision falls dramatically; ischaemia of the iris results in tissue damage with release of irritant autolytic products causing inflammatory and congestive signs — the typical acute glaucoma: a very hard, injected eye with a semi-dilated, non-reacting pupil and corneal oedema (19.10).

In the early stages the angle may open spontaneously, for example during sleep, and between attacks the eye may appear completely normal except for the narrow angle and shallow anterior chamber. Incomplete recovery may result in adhesion of parts of the iris root to the trabecular region causing a chronic obstruction to outflow. The intraocular pressure is controlled by systemic acetazolamide and topical pilocarpine in acute attacks. It is possible to prevent recurrence of the condition by creating an alternative path for aqueous flow through a hole in the peripheral iris by the use of surgery or laser.

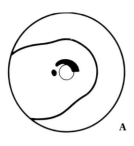

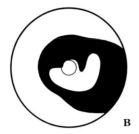

19.9 Visual field:
A early, B late

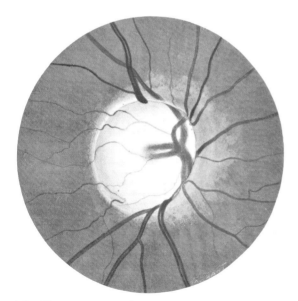

19.8 Glaucomatous cupping

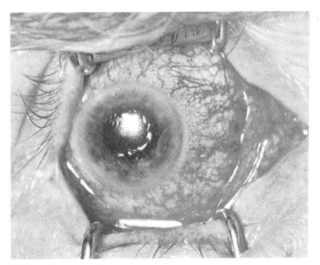

19.10 Acute closed angle glaucoma

20 *Abnormalities of ocular movements*

Deviation of the eyes from their normal position may be apparent only: a pseudostrabismus; an abnormality of muscle balance: a phoria; or a true lack of parallelism between the optic axes: a squint.

Pseudostrabismus

Pseudostrabismus, in which the visual axes appear not to be parallel, may be caused by prominent skin folds at the inner canthus, termed epicanthus (3.2).

Heterophoria

Normally accommodation and convergence are perfectly linked so that the movements of the two eyes bring the visual axes to the point of focus. In heterophoria this balance is lost and the eyes tend to converge or diverge too much for a given distance. No squint is present, but if one eye is covered it will be seen to have moved away from fixation when the cover is removed, returning quickly to take up fixation again. If the imbalance is in the vertical axis the patient tilts his head to restore the balance (ocular torticollis) (20.1).

Concomitant strabismus

In concomitant strabismus the angle of deviation remains approximately the same in all directions of gaze. Convergent squint, which may be familial, is the commonest type. The squint, at first intermittent, is usually noticed between the ages of one and two years, and may be precipitated by a systemic disease such as measles.

It is of the greatest importance that any child suspected of having a squint should be properly investigated as squint may be the presentation of a serious ocular or neurologic disorder. Untreated squint may lead to suppression of vision in one eye (amblyopia). Children under the age of ten have immature visual development and often suppress the central vision from one eye when squinting, to avoid diploplia. This decrease in vision may persist when the better eye is covered (squint-induced amblyopia).

The presence of a squint is confirmed by a cover test. The patient is asked to view an object, and the examiner occludes one eye and then the other. A squint is present if one eye shifts to take up fixation when its fellow eye is occluded (20.2A and 20.2B).

The ophthalmologist assesses the acuity, refraction and health of each eye as well as the state of binocular vision. It is important to exclude serious treatable ocular disorders such as retinoblastoma or paediatric cataract. Spectacles are prescribed when they decrease the angle of squint or when they improve vision. Amblyopia is treated by supervised occlusion of the better eye in children with potential for further visual maturation (i.e. under the age of 10). Orthoptic exercises may help to maintain binocular status.

Early squint surgery is indicated in the cases where other measures have failed to control the squint and early restoration of normal ocular alignment is likely to restore binocular fusion. Cosmetic squint surgery can be performed at any age provided amblyopia has been optimally treated and the squint has been fully assessed. Children under the age of ten with squints must be followed carefully to ensure they do not require spectacles or treatment for amblyopia (whether they have had surgery or not!).

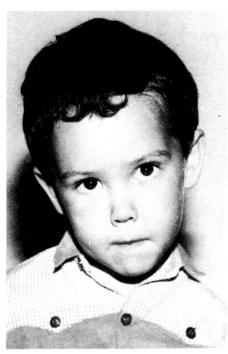

20.1 Ocular torticollis

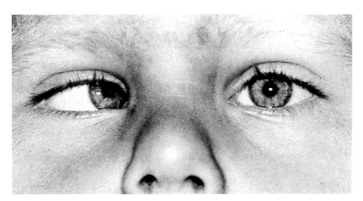

20.2A The right eye appears convergent when both eyes are open

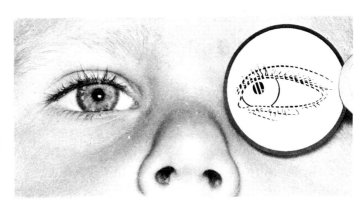

20.2B This is confirmed by the right eye shifting to take up fixation when the left eye is occluded

Abnormalities of ocular movements (cont.)

Paralytic strabismus

The angle of squint varies with the direction of gaze in incomitant squints. The commonest incomitant squints are paralysis affecting the sixth, third or fourth cranial nerves and internuclear ophthalmoplegia. Other causes of incomitant squint include dysthyroid eye disease, orbital trauma and myaesthenia gravis.

Paresis of an extraocular muscle results in limitation of movement of the affected eye in the direction of action of the muscle, with resultant diploplia. The separation of the images is greatest in the direction of action of the paretic muscle. It is important to establish the cause of paralytic and incomitant squints as they may be the presenting symptom of serious neurol-ogical or systemic disease. Simple diagnostic measures should not be overlooked (e.g. cardiac and vascular examination, identification of localising neurologic signs, blood glucose and measurement of erythrocyte sedimentation rate).

Sixth cranial nerve palsy presents with horizontal diploplia on looking towards the affected side. The eye on the affected side does not abduct past the straight ahead position (20.3). Third cranial nerve palsy presents with ptosis, mydriasis and an eye which is abducted and depressed (20.4).

Fourth cranial nerve palsy presents with vertical and torsional diploplia. The underaction of the superior oblique muscle is subtle.

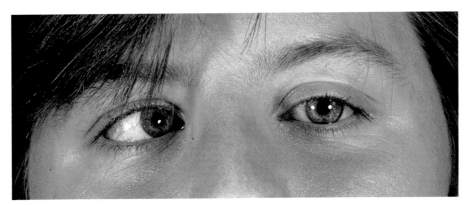

20.3   Left sixth nerve palsy with failure of left abduction

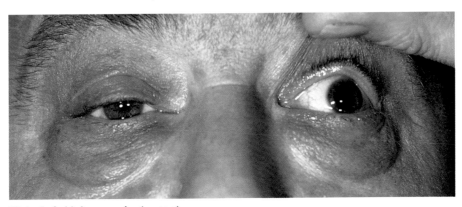

20.4   Left third nerve palsy (see text)

21 *Errors of refraction*

Errors of refraction are by far the commonest cause of defective vision. In order to see clearly in the distance parallel rays of light have to be brought to a focus on the retina by the optical components of the eye and if this is attained with the accommodation relaxed, the eye is said to be emmetropic (21.1).

Three main factors determine the refraction — the curvature of the cornea, the position and refractive power of the lens and the axial length of the eye. In spite of the variability in each of these factors in a normal population it is a remarkable fact that the majority of adults achieve emmetropia. The mechanism whereby the necessary adjustment of the three factors results in emmetropia is not yet understood but it seems certain that it is an active process, as a random combination of corneal curvature, lens power and axial length would result in a much wider spread of refractions than is observed.

Not all eyes achieve emmetropia and the relation between refractive power and axial length may be such that the image of a distant object is brought to a focus in front of the retina (myopia) or behind the retina (hypermetropia), or may not be completely clear in any position as in astigmatism.

In myopia (21.2) parallel rays are brought to a focus in front of the retina and need to be diverged by a minus (concave) lens for the image to be focused on the retina. Rays from objects closer to the eye are diverging and at one particular distance will be in focus so that the myope is said to be near-sighted. Myopia is usually the result of an increase in axial length and in the higher degrees this can cause stretching and thinning of the retina making the eye more susceptible to retinal detachment and degenerative changes at the posterior pole (21.4).

In hypermetropia (21.3), the eye tends to be smaller than normal so that rays from a distant object do not meet at the retina and a plus (convex) lens is required to provide the additional convergence. The hypermetrope can however increase the converging power of the lens by accommodating and may be able to bring a distant object into focus — hence the name far-sighted. In very small hypermetropic eyes, crowding of the nerve fibres as they enter the eye at the optic disc may give an appearance simulating papilloedema (21.5).

Astigmatism is a condition in which the refraction of the eye is not regular but varies in different axes so that a cylindrical lens has to be positioned in one axis to bring the refraction of the two axes to the same focus. Astigmatism may accompany myopia or hypermetropia.

Presbyopia (old sight) affects us all in middle age and is due to the inability of the aging lens to change its shape during accommodation. A young person, if he or she is emmetropic (or wearing a suitable correction), is able to focus an object 7 cm in front of the eye. This power of accommodation is progressively reduced with age so that at 40 years objects nearer than 25 cm cannot be seen clearly even when the eye is fully accommodated. 25 cm is a satisfactory distance for most close work, but once the near point recedes further, reading material has to be held further and further from the eye and plus lenses are needed for near work.

If the lens is removed from the eye (e.g. after cataract extraction), the eye becomes hypermetropic and the extra lens power has to be added either by spectacles, contact lenses, or the insertion of a small lens into the eye at the time of surgery.

Optical correction

Most refractive problems can be corrected simply and satisfactorily by spectacle lenses. Contact lenses act by providing a new artificial corneal curvature and have cosmetic and in some cases optical advantages. Newer materials and designs mean that the patient can choose between hard and soft contact lenses. Some soft lenses can be worn for weeks continuously, though their use is associated with an increased rate of infective keratitis. Contact lenses require meticulous cleaning, disinfection and storage.

Common problems with contact lenses include corneal hypoxia ('overwear') and intolerance of contact lens wear due to anterior segment inflammatory conditions. Microbial keratitis is a relatively uncommon sight-threatening complication.

The anterior corneal surface can be remodelled by surgery or laser to allow the myopic patient to achieve better vision without the use of spectacles or contact lenses. Radial keratotomy is the commonest corneal refractive procedure. Several radial cuts are made into the anaesthetised cornea away from the visual axis. This flattens the cornea and corrects low degrees of myopia (21.6). The surgical result is not altogether predictable for higher degrees of myopia, and there are risks attached to the procedure. Lasers have been used experimentally to remodel the anterior corneal surface to correct myopia, hypermetropia and astigmatism.

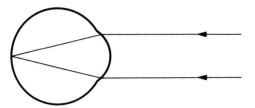

21.1   Emmetropia

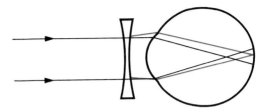

21.2   Myopia

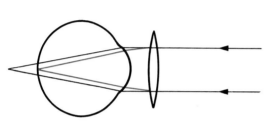

21.3   Hypermetropia

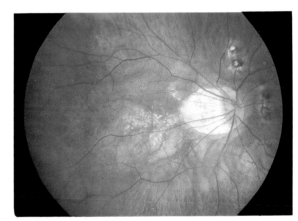

21.4   Degenerative myopic fundus

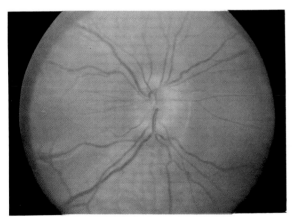

21.5   Pseudopapilloedema

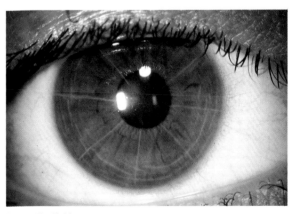

21.6   Radial keratotomy scars

22 *The normal fundus*

Seen ophthalmoscopically, the normal fundus varies within wide limits. What may be described as two very typical examples are seen in 22.1 and 22.2, the first as taken by a standard camera (at X 10) and the second by wide angle. The most prominent feature is the optic disc, round or slightly oval in shape, which marks the entrance of the optic nerve. It dips down slightly in the centre into a physiological cup which varies considerably in depth and configuration in different eyes, and from it the retinal vessels radiate, dividing dichotomously into innumerable branches as they spread over the fundus (22.2). Their walls are normally transparent and the blood column in the arteries appears a brighter red than that in the slightly purplish veins. Moreover, the arteries are narrower and show a slightly more brilliant bright streak than the veins, because the light is reflected partly from the convex cylindrical blood column and partly from the media of the walls.

The macula

The macula is the most important region of the fundus, since it subserves central vision. It lies some two disc diameters to the temporal side of the optic disc and somewhat below its centre. It is depicted in 22.3. It is usually slightly deeper in tint than the surrounding fundus, owing to the greater thickness of the subjacent choriocapillaris. In its centre is a small pit, the fovea, which normally appears as a bright reflex, since the light of the ophthalmoscope is reflected from its curved walls. The reflex varies considerably in shape and intensity, but the illustration shows one of the more simple and common appearances.

Cilio-retinal vessels

The pattern of the normal retinal vessels varies considerably and is of little clinical significance; but occasionally part of the retina is supplied by a vessel derived from the ciliary system. Such a vessel, usually an artery, is called a cilio-retinal vessel. Such vessels appear at the margin of the disc and curve over its edge to supply the adjacent retina. Commonly a vessel of this type goes to the macular region and, should the central retinal artery become blocked, macular vision may be preserved in this event by the unaffected cilio-retinal artery.

General pigmentation

The general pigmentation of the background of the fundus varies between individuals. If the pigment is deficient, the choroidal vessels may sometimes be seen; they are distinguished from the retinal vessels in that they have no central reflex, are broader and anastomose freely. In heavily pigmented people the fundus is a darker red, and if the retinal epithelium preponderates it shows a fine pigmented stippling, while if the choroidal pigment is dense in comparison with that of the retinal epithelium, the polygonal areas between the choroidal vessels appear darkly outlined, giving the appearance of a *tessellated* or *tigroid* fundus, seen in 22.4. A ring of pigment which may be complete but is usually partial surrounds the optic disc in many normal eyes.

In coloured patients the fundus background assumes a greenish colour which contrasts sharply with the optic disc. The retinal vessels also appear darker in such eyes (22.5).

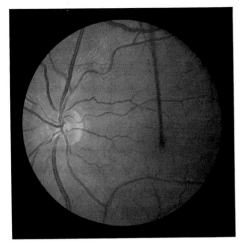

22.1A Fundus photo

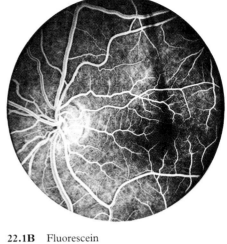

22.1B Fluorescein

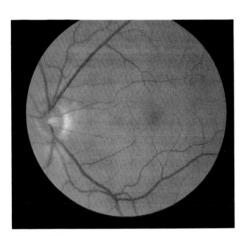

22.2 Wide angle picture of a normal fundus

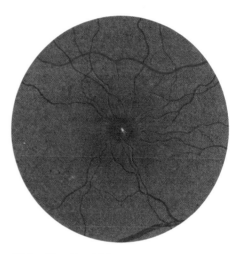

22.3 Macular region

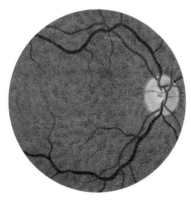

22.4 Tigroid fundus

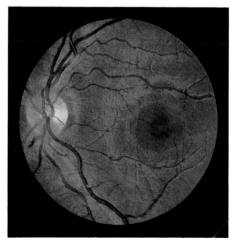

22.5 Negro fundus

23 Arteriosclerosis and hypertension

A diffuse degeneration of the media is an almost universal finding in the arteries of older patients, but the recognition of such changes in the retinal vessels is complicated by the hypertensive changes that so frequently accompany arteriosclerosis.

In the absence of hypertension the earliest changes are an increase in light reflex from the arterial wall and masking of the veins at the arterio-venous crossings. Normally it is possible to distinguish a vein through the overlying artery, but when the arterial wall becomes thickened, this is no longer possible. Later the arteries become more tortuous and show irregularities of calibre, well seen in 23.1. The irregularity is most marked near the disc and frequently the bloodstream is narrowed to a fine thread for a section of the vessel.

At the arterio-venous crossings the veins become nipped and deflected so as to meet the arteries more nearly at a right angle, and the peripheral section of the vein becomes engorged.

In later stages the arteries assume a 'copper-wire' or 'silver-wire' appearance due to the increased reflection of light from the vessel wall and haemorrhages and hard white exudates develop, particularly in the macular region (23.2).

Acute hypertensive retinopathy may appear particularly in young patients but is usually superimposed on arteriosclerotic changes. It is characterized by narrowing of the arterioles which may progress to partial or complete obliteration leading to areas of ischaemic infarction of the retina which can be recognized ophthalmoscopically as 'cotton-wool' spots (23.3). Aneurysmal dilatations and retinal haemorrhages are commonly present. In addition to the localized areas of oedema in the cotton-wool spots there may be some general swelling of the retina and optic disc, producing a picture similar to the papilloedema of raised intracranial pressure (23.4).

The exudates tend to follow the pattern of the nerve fibre layer and become arranged in a star configuration around the macula (23.5).

Fluorescein angiography demonstrates the arteriolar narrowing with tortuosity of the vessels and microaneurysm formation. Focal areas of capillary obliteration can be seen and in the later stages leakage of dye occurs from the abnormal retinal capillaries.

The picture of hypertensive retinopathy is one of the most dramatic in ophthalmology and is also of unusual importance from the point of view of general medicine, since it provides a clear and unequivocal view of the state of the arterioles and reflects particularly the condition of the vessels of corresponding size in the cerebral circulation.

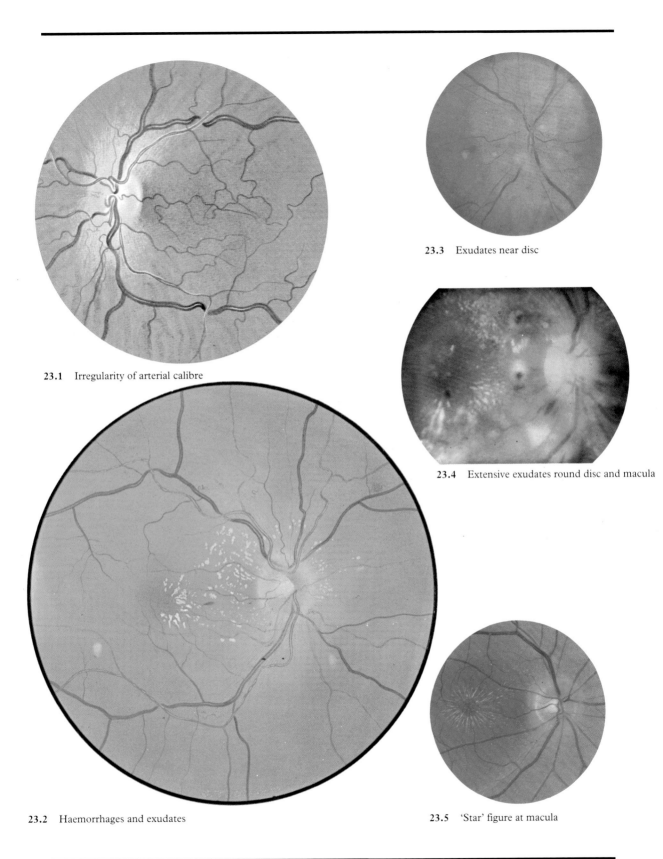

23.1 Irregularity of arterial calibre

23.2 Haemorrhages and exudates

23.3 Exudates near disc

23.4 Extensive exudates round disc and macula

23.5 'Star' figure at macula

24 *Arterial and venous occlusions*

Retinal arterial occlusion

Arterial occlusion of the central artery of the retina or one of its branches may be due to spasm, embolism or thrombosis, and unless the obstruction is removed within a few hours, permanent loss of function of that part of the retina supplied by the vessel will result. Atheromatous disease of the carotid vessels is the commonest cause of embolic central artery occlusion, while thrombosis may be the result of a true vasculitis or an incident in the course of retinal arteriosclerosis.

However the obstruction is caused, the sequence of events in the retina is the same. The larger arteries are extremely narrowed and the blood column, particularly in the veins, may be broken up into segments, which oscillate with the pulse waves. Meanwhile the retina becomes oedematous and loses its transparency, so that the whole fundus appears much paler then normal except for the macula, which shows up as a bright cherry-red spot standing out prominently against the light background. The disc is also pale. Treatment by the inhalation of amyl nitrite, the retrobulbar injection of acetylcholine, and other vasodilators should be instigated immediately. Vigorous massage of the globe or paracentesis of the anterior chamber may encourage the embolus to move to a more peripheral vessel and improve the retinal circulation. It is important to identify and treat potential sources of recurrent emboli such as cardiac valve disease, carotid arterial disease and arrythmias. The erythrocyte sedimentation rate should be measured, as giant cell arteritis can cause retinal arterial occlusion.

It is not uncommon to see a vessel supplying the macular region which is not a branch of the central retinal artery but a cilio-retinal artery derived from the short ciliary vessels. In such a case obstruction of the central artery will leave the retina supplied by the cilioretinal artery unaffected, thus preserving some central vision but with complete loss of the peripheral field.

After a few weeks the retina may regain its normal appearance although the vessels remain small and the disc pale.

24.1 shows the pale central area, with the bright-red spot at the macula and some fragmentation of the blood in the lower nasal vessels. Blockage of the inferior temporal branch is shown in 24.2. Here the pallor and narrowing of the vessels are confined to the lower temporal area.

Retinal vein obstruction

The central retinal vein or a tributary of the vein may become occluded as a result of generalized vascular disease in older patients or more rarely from inflammatory lesions in younger patients. Modern methods of investigation such as fluorescein angiography have shown that central retinal vein occlusion can be subdivided into two broad categories. The more serious condition (haemorrhagic retinopathy) is accompanied by severe retinal oedema due to closure of the capillary circulation. The vision is severely depressed and the chances of visual recovery are poor. The retinal ischaemia stimulates fragile new vessel proliferation on the retina which may lead to vitreous haemorrhage from rupture of the vessels. The fundus picture is characterized by marked swelling of the disc, great engorgement of the retinal veins and a large number of retinal haemorrhages both superficial and deep (24.3A). The fluorescein appearance of a typical central retinal vein occlusion is shown in 24.3B.

The other type of occlusion is characterized by venous stasis without capillary obliteration. Again there is some swelling of the disc with engorgement of the veins and oedema of the posterior pole. The haemorrhagic aspect is however less marked and the haemorrhages which do occur are found more peripherally in the fundus. Vision is less severely affected than in the haemorrhagic type and considerable recovery can be expected (24.4).

The occluded vein may recanalize in time and new collateral vessels form so that the circulation is restored, the oedema subsides and the haemorrhages are absorbed. In those cases in which there has been retinal ischaemia new vessels may form on the iris and in the angles of the anterior chamber weeks or months later. The vessels in the angle stimulate the formation of peripheral anterior synechiae which close off the drainage of aqueous and result in an intractable form of secondary glaucoma. Peripheral retinal laser photocoagulation dramatically reduces the incidence of complications of retinal ischaemia following central or branch retinal vein occlusion. These complications include vitreous haemorrhage and painful rubeotic glaucoma. It is important to identify and treat systemic conditions which predispose retinal vein occlusion (e.g. diabetes, hypertension, hyperlipidaemia or cigarette smoking).

In some cases a branch vein may become occluded at the point where it is crossed by an artery giving the picture of branch vein thrombosis (24.5).

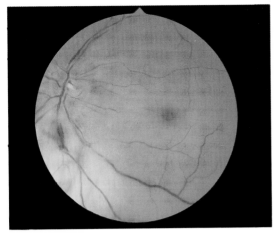

24.1 Occlusion of central retinal artery

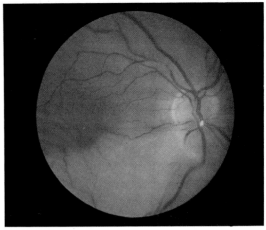

24.2 Inferior temporal branch artery occlusion

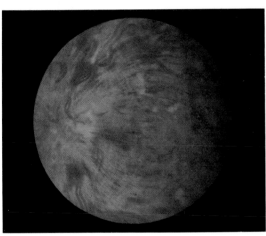

24.3A Central vein occlusion major

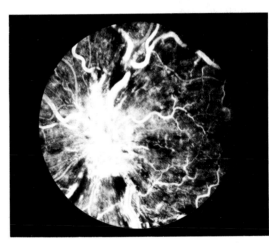

24.3B Fluorescein picture

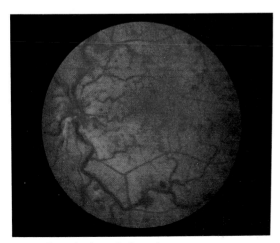

24.4 Central vein occlusion minor

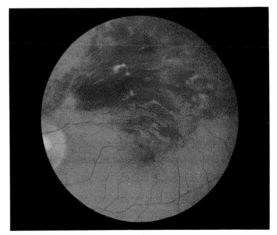

24.5 Branch vein occlusion

25 *Diabetic retinopathy*

It is well established that the incidence of diabetic retinopathy increases with the duration of the diabetes and the retinal lesions may progress in spite of an apparently well controlled blood sugar level. The disease is always bilateral but frequently affects one eye more than the other.

Background retinopathy

The earliest sign of diabetic retinopathy is an engorgement of the veins. This is followed by degenerative changes in the walls of the terminal vessels particularly on the venous side with the formation of micro-aneurysms. The earliest signs ophthalmoscopically are small dot haemorrhages and hard exudates scattered around the posterior pole (25.1). Fluorescein angiography shows a much more dramatic picture demonstrating the vascular abnormalities (in particular the micro-aneurysms) in the early pictures and marked late leakage of dye from them. These changes are known as background retinopathy and are asymptomatic. From here the disease tends to progress along two pathways: one exudative and the other vasoproliferative.

Exudative

Here there is increasing disease of small vessels at the posterior pole resulting in progressive hard exudate formation with accompanying dot retinal haemorrhages (25.2A). Central vision dimimshes and there may be small minute field defects coinciding with the hard exudates. If the macula itself is involved, permanent loss of central vision occurs. Fluorescein angiography demonstrates profuse leakage from the vascular abnormalities related to the exudates (25.2B).

Treatment is most effective when given at an early stage of the disease. Argon laser or Xenon photocoagulation should be applied to the vascular abnormalities around the macula concentrating on the areas above and temporal to the macula but avoiding the papillo-macular bundle as much as possible.

Wet maculopathy is the term used for chronic oedema of the macula with the minimum of haemorrhages and hard exudate. There is a marked fall in central vision which may fluctuate in intensity. Fluorescein angiography demonstrates a diffuse leakage of dye from the small vessels surrounding the macula (25.3). Argon laser treatment may be helpful here if applied in a C around the macula with the open side facing the disc.

Ischaemic maculopathy is a severe form of diabetic retinopathy with a profound fall in central vision. Ophthalmoscopically no gross lesion is seen at the macula apart from a few haemorrhages and exudates. Fluorescein angiography however shows a marked lack of filling of small vessels around the macula (25.4). There may be some late leakage of dye from surrounding vessels. There is no treatment for this condition unfortunately.

Mixed forms of these retinopathies occur with varying components of exudates, ischaemia and oedema.

Proliferative retinopathy

New vessels may be formed anywhere in the fundus. The main tendency is from the disc and around the posterior pole. Proliferative retinopathy follows chronic retinal ischaemic changes. These changes are asymptomatic and may be difficult to see with the ophthalmoscope. Fluorescein angiography delineates

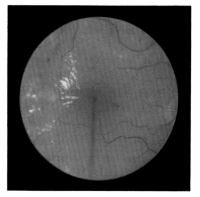

25.1 Background diabetic retinopathy

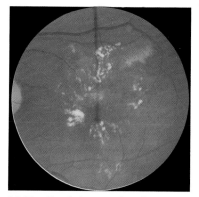

25.2A Exudative maculopathy

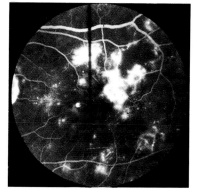

25.2B Exudative maculopathy (fluorescein)

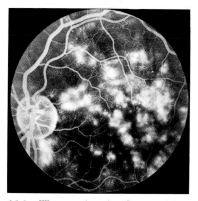

25.3 Wet maculopathy (fluorescein)

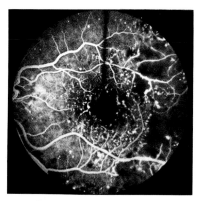

25.4 Ischaemic macula (fluorescein)

these vessels well, showing very early leakage of dye from them (25.5). Initially they lie flat on the surface of the retina but there is usually an accompanying change in the vitreous with collapse of the gel and partial posterior detachment. The areas still in contact with the retina provide bridges for the vessels to grow forwards on to the posterior surface of the vitreous away from the retina (25.6). At this stage there are no symptoms, but later on there is a tendency for these vessels to proliferate, fracture and bleed causing a retrogel haemorrhage. If this is massive in degree the vitreous is penetrated and a true vitreous haemorrhage occurs. This produces dramatic sudden loss of vision. The blood usually slowly clears from the vitreous but in some cases becomes an organised vitreous haemorrhage with longstanding loss of vision. The new vessels tend to proliferate and bleed repeatedly and after each bleed there is a reparative process involving fibrosis. Fibrous bridges then develop between different areas of the retina forming very firm attachments. Later on there is contraction of these membranes giving rise to retinal traction which will cause distortion of central vision if present at the macula. Progressive traction will cause retinal tears and traction retinal detachment (25.7). The treatment of choice is pan-retinal photocoagulation at an early stage in the disease. Peripheral retinal photocoagulation can be performed with Xenon Arc light or laser. This causes involution of the new vessels within a few days if adequate treatment has been applied. Continuing growth of new vessels should be treated by further photocoagulation to the retinal periphery. An organised vitreous haemorrhage if it persists for up to six months without resolution can be successfully removed by vitrectomy. If no view of the retina can be obtained it is advisable to carry out a dynamic ultrasound B scan to see if there is any retinal detachment. Traction retinal detachments are difficult to treat and involve complicated vitreous surgery with moderate results only.

There can of course be mixed degrees of all the retinopathies described and they should be treated appropriately.

In view of the lack of symptoms in early forms of retinopathy and because the results of treatment in patients presenting late are so bad, it is better to screen longstanding diabetics regularly for the retinopathy. This should be done by a trained ophthalmologist using careful ophthalmoscopy through a dilated pupil. Any retinopathy detected should then be promptly treated.

Screening for diabetic retinopathy

Routine ophthalmic screening should begin at presentation in patients whose disease is diagnosed after the age of 30; screening of younger patients should begin no later than five years after diabetes has been diagnosed. Screening should be performed by an experienced observer after the pupil has been dilated.

Proliferative retinopathy occurs more commonly in patients who have had diabetes for ten or more years. The frequency of follow up is determined by the severity of retinopathy. Urgent referral to an ophthalmologist is advised for any diabetic patient with new vessels anywhere in the fundus (especially the optic disc), exudative retinopathy threatening the fovea, or with a recent drop in vision.

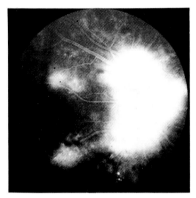

25.5 Vasoproliferative retinopathy
(fluorescein)

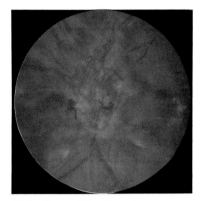

25.6 Vasoproliferative retinopathy

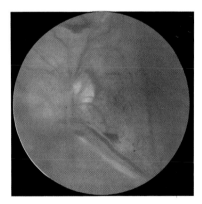

25.7 Traction detachment with diabetes

26 *The fundus in blood diseases*

Retinal changes are frequently seen in association with diseases of the blood.

Anaemia

Any severe anaemia may produce retinal changes of the type shown in 26.1. Some engorgement of the veins is common and flame-shaped haemorrhages with a pale centre occur. 'Cotton-wool' spots may be present.

Loss of vision may follow severe haemorrhage, particularly when the bleeding is recurrent. It is more likely to occur after haematemesis, renal haemorrhage or haemoptysis rather than after acute traumatic haemorrhage.

Leukaemia

Dilatation of the veins and papilloedema are common in severe cases of polycythaemia and leukaemia. In the early stages of leukaemia the retinal vessels are grossly dilated and haemorrhages are present (26.2). In the late stages the retina looks pale and the disc swollen due to leucocytic infiltration (26.3).

Macroglobulinaemia

Macroglobulinaemia is one of a group of diseases in which abnormal globulins are present in the plasma. The systemic symptoms are vague, with weakness, anorexia and haemorrhages from mucous membranes. The ocular changes, like the systemic changes, are due largely to an increase in the viscosity of the blood.

Venous congestion is the earliest sign and progresses to gross venous engorgement, retinal haemorrhages and congestion of the optic disc, giving an appearance rather like that of a venous thrombosis.

Sickle cell disease

Eye complications are seen in two of the genetic types of sickle cell disease: SS and SC. It is thought that the main aetiological factor is the red cells becoming elongated into a sickle form under conditions of reduced oxygen tension. The abnormal cells therefore become impacted in the capillaries at such sites as spleen, intestine, lung, kidneys, joints and bones. In the eye the changes are due to stasis and obstruction of the small vessels in the periphery of the retina. The earliest signs here are sunburst spots and salmon patches, shown in 26.4 A & B.

Capillary infarction in the retinal periphery causes chronic retinal ischaemia which, in turn, can cause peripheral new-vessel formation ('sea-fans') (26.5). It can be seen on the fluorescein angiogram that there is almost total absence of filling peripheral to these lesions (26.6). After their development the disease may follow two courses: either there is spontaneous thrombosis and resolution of the sea-fans, or progressive development of new vessels and fibrous tissue. Contraction produces pre-retinal and vitreous haemorrhages and eventually retinal tears and traction detachments. At the moment it is debatable whether laser treatment helps the disease.

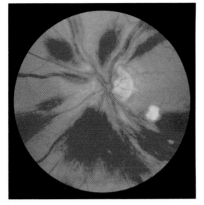

26.1 Anaemic retinopathy

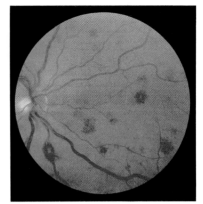

26.2 Early leukaemic retinopathy

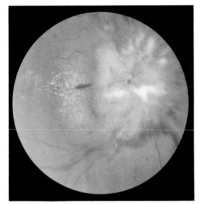

26.3 Disc infiltration in late leukaemia

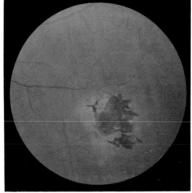

26.4A Sickle cell 'sun burst' spot

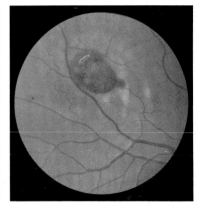

26.4B Sickle cell 'salmon patch'

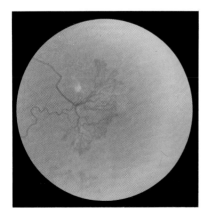

26.5 Sickle cell 'sea fan'

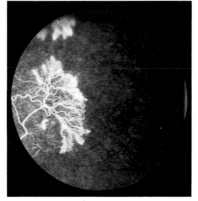

26.6 Sickle cell 'sea fan' (fluorescein)

27 *Miscellaneous conditions involving the retina*

Haemangiomatosis

Haemangiomatosis of the retina is always part of a wider syndrome in which angiomatous lesions are found in the skin, brain and other organs (von Hippel-Lindau's disease). The clinical appearances are very variable and may range from a single angioma (27.1) with its greatly dilated afferent and efferent vessels to a gross exudative retinal detachment with many enormously dilated vessels, haemorrhages and exudates involving the whole fundus. Secondary glaucoma and degeneration of the eye may follow. It is difficult to treat but cryotherapy or laser treatment to localised areas of tumour formation has met with some success.

Exudative retinitis or Coats' disease

This condition is seen in children and young adults, usually males. It is normally uni-ocular and is insidious in onset and progress. In the early stages flecks of deep retinal exudate appear scattered widely over the fundus which as the disease progresses conglomerate to form a subretinal mass (27.2). Coats originally described changes in the blood vessels, especially in the veins, as characteristic of the later stages, but these are not always seen. It is now felt that the earliest changes are telangiectasia of the small vessels of the retina (27.3A) which tend to increase in size leading to small aneurysm formation, superficial haemorrhages, and considerable fatty exudation. Fluorescein angiography delineates these vessels nicely and shows considerable late leakage (27.3B). In some cases the condition appears to be self-limiting, although an organised area remains in the fundus indefinitely. In the majority of cases, however, the subretinal exudate leads to the development of a retinal detachment with much gliosis. Progressive exudation may lead to complicated glaucoma and loss of the eye. There is a rare adult form of the disease with development of capillary telangiectasia and exudation. If this involves the macular region central vision is reduced. However, the disease has a much more limited course than that in the juvenile form and can be treated with the Argon laser.

Eales' disease

Eales' disease is a chronic retinal periphlebitis occurring in young adults, particularly men, and is characterised by recurrent vitreous haemorrhages. The condition starts as a patch of inflammation in and around the vessel wall, showing as a greyish fluffy exudate which may obscure the vein. Scattered lesions of this type may be found all round the periphery of the fundus. Usually both eyes are affected, one more than the other in the early stages of the disease. 27.4 shows the exudates well and fluorescein angiography demonstrates leakage from the affected vessels. Retinal haemorrhages accompany the acute phase and frequently the blood penetrates into the vitreous, completely obscuring the fundus and causing sudden loss of vision. This is usually the symptom which brings the patient for advice. In the early attacks the vitreous may clear completely, but later organisation of the recurrent haemorrhages may take place, giving rise to retinitis proliferans — this may undergo fibrous retraction giving rise to retinal traction, tears and detachments. The aetiology is obscure.

Retinal vasculitis

This is a heading for a group of diseases similar to the above where there are signs of inflammation related to retinal veins, arterioles or capillaries. Venous and arteriolar sheathing or occlusion may be seen. Small retinal haemorrhages and cotton-wool spots accompany capillary involvement. The vasculitides vary in severity and many are accompanied by inflammation elsewhere in the eye (e.g. uveitis) or elsewhere systemically.

Sarcoidosis, Behcet's disease, systemic lupus (SLE) and polyarteritis nodosa (PAN) may all cause retinal vasculitis, although the aetiology is obscure in many cases. A number of intracellular infectious agents are associated with retinal vasculitis, often with characteristic retinal manifestations. HIV, cytomegalovirus, and other herpetic viruses can all affect the retina in this way, and are discussed in the chapter on the ocular manifestation of AIDS. Retinal vasculitis tends to remit after varying periods. Systemic immunosuppression is used with varying degrees of success when sight is threatened by retinal vasculitis.

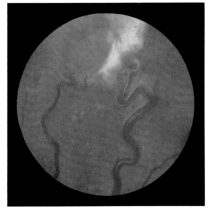

27.1 Single haemangioma

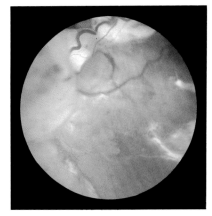

27.2 Coats' exudative retinopathy

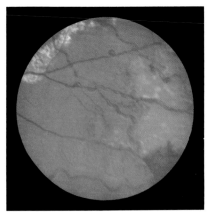

27.3A Retinal telangiectasia

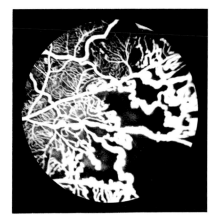

27.3B Telangiectasia fluorescein

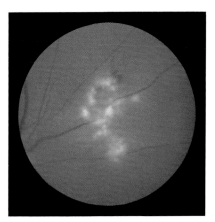

27.4 Perivascular exudates

28 *Choroiditis*

Inflammatory lesions of the choroid and retina may be divided into two broad groups according to the clinical appearances: disseminated choroiditis in which multiple lesions, usually small, are scattered over the fundus, and focal chorioretinitis in which one or a few larger lesions are found in one area of the fundus. Two of the more common conditions causing focal lesions are described in the next section.

Disseminated choroiditis

Disseminated choroiditis results from multiple foci of infection reaching the choroid from the bloodstream via the short ciliary arteries. The lesions tend to occur in the equatorial and peripheral areas of the retina, and in the acute stage are characterized by multiple small yellowish-white fluffy spots. As healing takes place the centre of the lesions becomes pale and atrophic and surrounded by accumulation of pigment (28.1).

Congenital syphilis is the commonest cause of disseminated choroiditis, and the lesions may vary in size in individual cases from the fine pin-point yellow and black spots of the typical 'pepper and salt' fundus (28.2) to much larger disseminated lesions. The condition is usually recognized on routine ophthalmoscopy when it is inactive, but recurrences sometimes occur with an interstitial keratitis.

Rubella may cause a retinopathy in addition to congenital cataract and produces a picture somewhat similar to the pepper and salt fundus of congenital syphilis (28.3). The condition has to be distinguished from retinitis pigmentosa which it also resembles but fortunately it is not progressive.

Miliary tuberculosis may cause scattered yellowish areas of choroiditis, and this is most often seen in cases of tuberculous meningitis (28.4).

Septic emboli from any focus of infection can cause a similar picture, but it is often difficult to find the primary source.

In patients whose immunological responses are reduced as a result of disease or treatment with immuno-suppressive drugs, opportunist infections may reach the eye and fungal infections in particular seem to have a predilection for the retina and the vitreous. Although the initial lesions are in the retina (28.5), invasion of the vitreous results in an endophthalmitis with fluffy balls of fungus visible ophthalmoscopically. The diagnosis is confirmed by vitreous biopsy and vitrectomy helps to remove fungus from the eye.

Histoplasmosis

This fungus, *Histoplasmosis capsulatum,* is endemic in large areas of North America and although absolute proof is still lacking, the epidemiological evidence is so convincing that the relationship between systemic infection and a particular ocular condition must be assumed. The primary infection, which is usually sub-clinical, results from inhalation of the spores and the formation of granulomas in the lung. It is thought that haematogenous spread results in the organisms reaching the choroid where they cause small foci of inflammation. At this stage the condition causes no symptoms but the small punched out scars adjacent to the optic disc and in the retinal periphery are frequently seen on routine examination of patients in endemic areas.

For reasons which are not clear, one of these lesions becomes active after many years and stimulates new vessel formation under the retina particularly in the macular area. Bleeding from the new vessels (28.6) results in sudden loss of vision and the subsequent scar which forms leaves a permanent visual impairment.

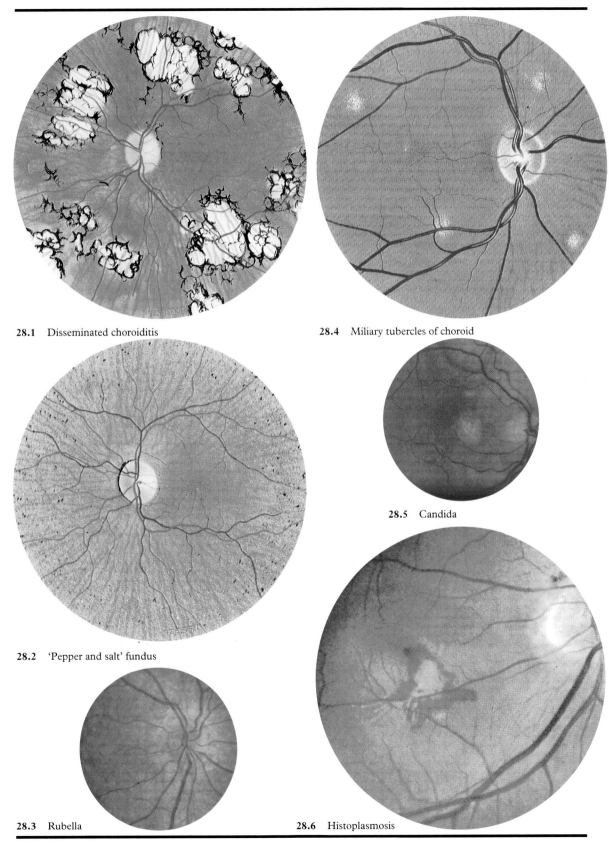

28.1 Disseminated choroiditis

28.4 Miliary tubercles of choroid

28.5 Candida

28.2 'Pepper and salt' fundus

28.3 Rubella

28.6 Histoplasmosis

29 *Toxoplasmosis and toxocariasis*

Toxoplasmosis

Although the toxoplasma organism was first discovered in 1908 by Nicolle and Manceaux its role as a pathogen in man was not recognized until thirty years later, when it was found to be the cause of a congenital disease characterized by bilateral choroidoretinitis and various systemic manifestations (29.1).

The organism is an intracellular protozoan parasite, and surveys have shown that it is a common infection of domestic and wild animals in most regions of the world. Serologic surveys have shown that human infection is very common, although most cases are subclinical. Some acute infections are accompanied by fever and lymphadenopathy. Ocular involvement is uncommon in acquired cases except in patients who are severely immunocompromised. However, a focal chorioretinitis identical in appearance to that seen in congenital toxoplasmosis does occur in children and young adults without any history of systemic disease but with serological evidence of past infection with toxoplasmosis. The organism has been recovered from such eyes and the condition responds to specific antitoxoplasmic treatment.

The explanation for this is that nearly all cases of toxoplasmic chorioretinitis affecting immunocompetent children and adults are the result of a recurrence of congenital infection. Unless the lesion involves the macula it will not be discovered in childhood, and it is only when a recurrence occurs that the symptoms of blurred vision and floating spots draw attention to the condition.

On examination there may be some anterior uveal reaction with keratic precipitates, flare and cells in the aqueous; the vitreous is hazy and fundus examination will show an active lesion at the edge of an old pigmented scar. These lesions are usually at the posterior pole in the region of the macula, disc or main vessels, but sometimes they are more peripherally sited (29.2 and 29.3). An old scar may also be found in the other eye.

These recurrences occur most frequently between the ages of 15 and 25, but their cause is unknown. Occasionally a history of recent injury to the eye is obtained, and sometimes there appears to be some relationship with stress or intercurrent infection. Recurrences may occur in pregnancy, giving rise to fear that the foetus may be affected. This fear is groundless, as it is known that foetal infection only occurs when the mother contracts the infection during pregnancy. Once she has developed circulating antibodies, spread of infection via the bloodstream to the foetus is extremely unlikely.

Diagnosis of toxoplasmic chorioretinitis in the adult depends on a focal lesion adjacent to an old scar and positive serological tests for toxoplasmosis. Previous toxoplasmosis infection can be demonstrated by finding specific serum antibodies directed against this organism in any titre. A high titre suggests recent infection, but there is no particular titre which is 'significant' in the diagnosis of toxoplasma retinitis. The absence of serum antibodies to toxoplasmosis makes the diagnosis unlikely, but do not exclude it as the organism has been recovered from the eyes of patients in whom such serum antibodies have been absent.

Toxocariasis

Small children sometimes become infected with the dog roundworm, *Toxocara canis*. The eggs are ingested and develop into larvae which migrate throughout the body. If a larva enters the eye it can cause a severe granulomatous reaction and produce a raised lesion at the posterior pole (29.4) or in the region of the ciliary body (29.5). Some degree of eosinophilia is usually present, and intradermal injection of an antigen made from the worm gives an immediate reaction in infected patients.

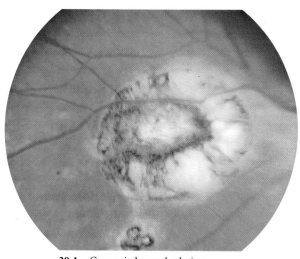

29.1 Congenital macular lesion

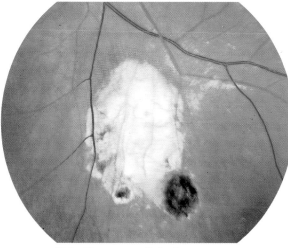

29.2 Recurrence of infection

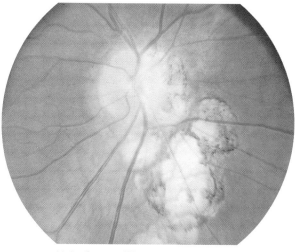

29.3 Juxtapapilliary choroiditis

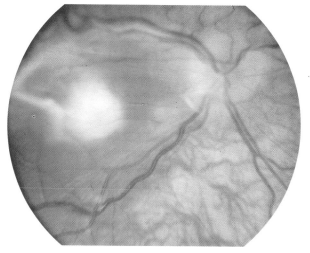

29.4 Toxocariasis

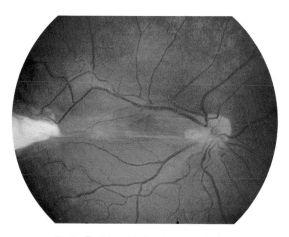

29.5 Peripheral lesion in toxocariasis

30 *Optic disc changes*

Drusen

Pale warty excrescences on the disc are not uncommonly seen, and represent a degenerative condition of the disc (30.1A). Their main importance is in the differential diagnosis of papilloedema. Fluorescein fundus photography provides an elegant means of differentiation, as drusen do not show any staining (30.1B), but in papilloedema a long-lasting fluorescence of the disc is present.

Pseudopapilloedema

This congenital variation from the normal appearance of the optic disc is found almost exclusively in small, hypermetropic eyes. It is caused by a heaping up of the nerve fibres combined with an excess of neuroglial tissue, causing the disc to project forward, sometimes to a considerable extent. As seen in 30.2, the entire disc is swollen with a greyish and somewhat ill-defined margin. The vessels are of normal calibre and appearance but bend in a curve as they pass from the swollen disc to the retina.

It is important to notice that venous engorgement, haemorrhages and exudates are never present. Frequently the vision cannot be corrected to the normal standard in these cases.

Papilloedema and optic neuritis

The importance of establishing a diagnosis of papilloedema cannot be overestimated. The fully developed condition is not easily misinterpreted, but minor degrees of swelling may be very difficult to diagnose.

Papilloedema is essentially a passive oedema due to raised intracranial pressure, the first evidence of which is an increased redness of the disc with some blurring of the margins, particularly of its upper and lower parts. The physiological cup becomes filled in and some sheathing of the vessels may be noticed. The veins become congested and the swelling of the disc increases. At this stage the whole margin of the disc becomes indistinct and flame-shaped haemorrhages and exudates begin to appear. In the fully developed condition, shown in 30.3, the disc can be seen to be considerably raised above the level of the surrounding retina; the veins are engorged and the vessels dip sharply down to the retina, losing their light reflex as they bend away from the observer.

The oedema spreads to the surrounding retina, particularly towards the macula, and may produce a partial macular star.

The appearance of an optic neuritis is very similar to that of papilloedema and the differential diagnosis depends essentially on the absence of raised intracranial pressure and the symptomatology. Papilloedema may have very little effect on central vision or the peripheral field, but in optic neuritis the loss of vision is marked and may precede the changes at the disc.

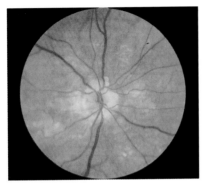
30.1A Drusen of optic disc

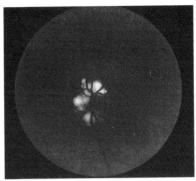
30.1B Autofluorescence of disc drusen

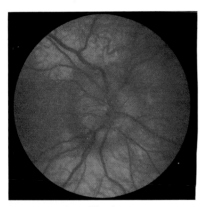
30.2 Pseudopapilloedema

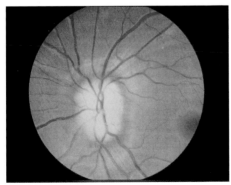
A

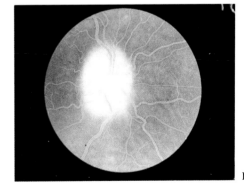
B

30.3 Papilloedema (**A**), with fluorescein angiogram (**B**) Showing leakage

30 *Optic disc changes (cont.)*

Optic atrophy

Optic atrophy may follow swelling of the disc or may arise without preceding oedema or inflammation.

The disc is very pale and shows up clearly against the surrounding fundus. The main retinal vessels are narrowed and some degree of cupping is present, due simply to atrophy of the nerve bundles. The lamina cribrosa is often clearly seen (30.4).

The atrophy may be limited to one portion of the disc only, as for example the temporal pallor following an optic neuritis in which the papillomacular bundle of fibres is particularly affected.

Two important treatable causes of optic atrophy are giant cell arteritis and mechanical compression of the anterior visual pathway (optic nerve, chiasm or optic tract). The site and progression of compressive lesions causing optic atrophy may be deduced from the patient's visual fields.

Ischaemic optic neuropathy

Anterior ischaemic optic neuropathy is a condition in which occlusion of the branches of the posterior ciliary arteries which supply the optic disc results in infarction of the disc and sudden loss of vision. Mild swelling of the disc occurs (30.5) sometimes with flame shaped haemorrhages.

It is important to distinguish between those cases due to atherosclerotic changes and those due to giant-cell arteritis (temporal arteritis). In the latter condition the visual loss is more severe and the patients have evidence of systemic disease such as myalgias and tenderness over the temporal arteries. The crucial test is the erythrocyte sedimentation rate which is always elevated above 40 mm/hr in giant-cell arteritis. This test must be done immediately if the condition is suspected and treatment started with high doses of corticosteroids to prevent the other eye becoming affected and resulting in bilateral blindness. The diagnosis of arteritic ischaemic optic neuropathy may, in many cases, be confirmed histologically by temporal artery biopsy.

Myopic crescent

The thinning and stretching of the posterior half of the globe in high myopia results in the exposure of a crescent of choroid and sclera round the optic disc (30.6).

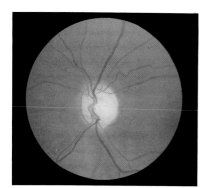

30.4 Optic atrophy

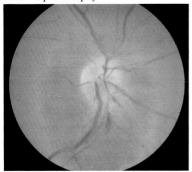

30.5 Anterior ischaemic optic neuropathy

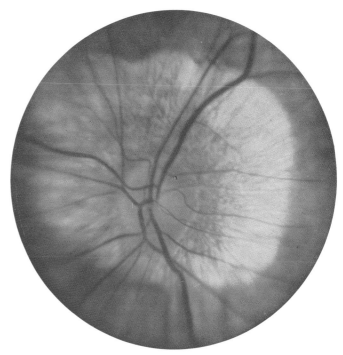

30.6 Myopic crescent

31 *Congenital anomalies of the fundus*

Oculocutaneous albinism

Albinism is congenital and may have an X-linked or recessive inheritance. Examination of freshly plucked hair bulbs for their ability to produce pigment when incubated with tyrosine has shown two broad biochemical types. Good pigment production suggests that tyrosinase is present in the melanocytes and such cases have a better prognosis than tyrosine negative patients in whom some vital component of the melanin pathway is lacking.

The eyebrows and lashes are usually white; this, combined with narrowing of the palpebral fissures to decrease the amount of light entering the eyes, presents a characteristic clinical appearance. The associated rapid horizontal or rotatory nystagmus may be due to poor central fixation. The iris is a pink-grey colour and in the pupil a red reflex can be seen due to light penetrating the sclera, traversing the depigmented choroid and illuminating the fundus. Fairly high refractive errors are common and vision is always poor, partly due to the scattering of light in the eye and partly due to the poor development and function of the macula in this condition. As shown in 31.1, the whole fundus is pale and the individual retinal and choroidal vessels show up clearly against the white sclera. The patients are always photophobic and much can be done to help them by providing dark glasses or tinted contact lenses with an artificial pupil.

Ocular albinism in which the defective pigmentation is mainly confined to the eye is also inherited as an X-linked or autosomal recessive trait and the ocular features are similar but less marked than those of the oculocutaneous form.

Coloboma

Colobomata are the result of imperfect closure of the foetal cleft of the optic vesicle in embryonic life, and on the extent of this imperfection will depend the extent of the coloboma. It may involve singly or together the iris, ciliary body, choroid, retina and optic nerve.

31.2 is a fundus photograph of a typical coloboma of the retina and choroid. Where the tissues are lacking the sclera shows up as a white area, the gap being bridged by thin, poorly differentiated tissue which may contain some retinal vessels. There is a scotoma in the visual field corresponding to, although usually smaller than, the defective area. Other congenital abnormalities are frequently present.

Opaque nerve fibres

Medullation of the optic fibres starts centrally, and at birth has normally reached a level immediately behind the lamina cribrosa, where the process stops. Sometimes, however, the process continues after birth (so that the condition is not truly congenital) and the appearance shown in 31.3 is produced.

The nerve fibres, which are normally transparent, appear brilliantly white and opaque against the red background of the fundus, and their arcuate course from the disc over the macular region can be clearly traced. The retinal vessels are partly obscured.

Vision is little affected, although there is a partial scotoma corresponding to the area involved.

Hole in the optic disc

In this condition an outpouching of the secondary optic vesicle produces a crater-like hole in the optic disc. The hole is usually oval in shape with the long axis vertical and it may vary in depth from a millimetre or so to a centimetre. It appears bluish-grey in colour, an optical effect probably due to shadows thrown on the floor of the pit (31.4). Pathological examination shows that the hole is lined by rudimentary retinal tissue. Retinal vessels sometimes enter the pit and descend to cross the floor before rising and continuing over the disc.

Slight degrees of the deformity produce no symptoms, but field defects and serous detachment of the central retina have been reported in association with larger craters.

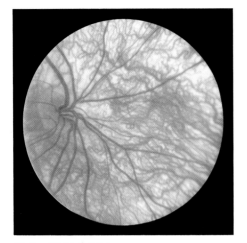

31.1 Albino fundus

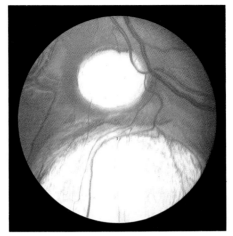

31.2 Coloboma of choroid

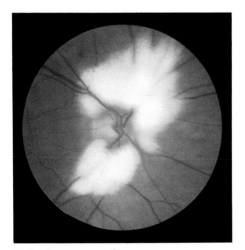

31.3 Opaque nerve fibres

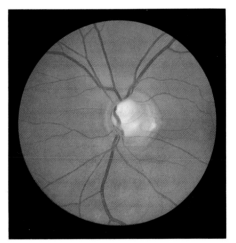

31.4 Congenital pit

32 *Trauma to the posterior segment*

Trauma to the eye may be roughly divided into concussion injuries and perforating injuries; whereas the fundus appearances naturally vary considerably, some typical changes may occur in each group.

Concussion injuries

These injuries follow blows on the eye from large objects such as a fist or tennis ball. The shock-wave travels through the fluid media of the eye and produces its main effects at the posterior pole. The retina, and in particular the macular region, like all highly developed tissue, is more susceptible to damage than the choroid. Comparatively trivial blows with little external evidence of injury may cause permanent macular lesions with diminished central vision — a good reason for giving a guarded prognosis in all ocular injuries.

Commotio retinae

Commotio retinae is the term used for oedema of the macular region following a concussion injury. The retina at the posterior pole becomes slightly opaque and has a milky sheen, the macula showing as a bright red spot (32.1). The oedema subsides but is often followed by pigmentary or cystic macular changes. The latter give the appearance of a sharply defined 'hole' at the macula (32.2); but microscopic examination has shown that the condition is really cystic. Central vision is markedly affected.

In more severe cases of concussion injury the choroid may be torn, as shown in 32.3, the tears appearing as yellowish streaks with some pigment disturbance at the edges, roughly concentric with the optic disc.

Retinal tears may also occur in such injuries and they are very likely to be followed by detachment. This complication will be described in a later section. Frequently, vitreous haemorrhages obscure the fundus picture in the more severe injuries and the extent of the retinal and choroidal damage can only be assessed when the haemorrhage has been absorbed.

Solar burn

Eclipse blindness is the result of a solar burn of the retina caused by looking directly at the sun (32.4). The retinal oedema shown here is later replaced by a discrete pigmented scar, sometimes with considerable reduction of central vision.

Perforating injuries

The grosser penetrating wounds caused by large objects usually cause such disorganization of the eye that the fundus cannot be seen, but frequently a small metallic foreign body may penetrate the globe, apparently causing remarkably little disturbance. The patient may feel little or no pain and unless the anterior chamber is lost or the lens injured, or haemorrhage takes place in the eye, the sight may not be immediately affected. It is not uncommon for the presence of the foreign body to be unsuspected for days, weeks or even years, until visual changes bring the patient for examination.

The amount of damage caused by the entry of the foreign body depends on its size and route. In hammer-and-chisel injuries, in which a small flake from the hammer-head flies back into the eye, the fragment usually penetrates the cornea, crosses the anterior chamber and goes through the iris or pupil and the lens. It may, however, enter at the limbus and pass through the zonule of the lens into the vitreous chamber. Its subsequent course depends on its propulsive force, but frequently it comes to rest embedded in the retina near the posterior pole.

32.5 shows such a foreign body embedded in the retina with consequent pigmentary changes; the vitreous disturbance caused by its passage is clearly seen. Optic atrophy may follow blunt or perforating eye injuries.

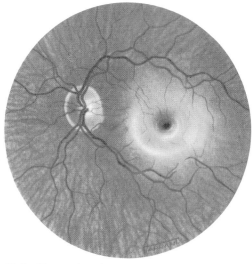

32.1 Commotio retinae

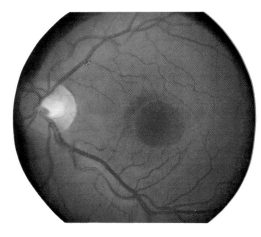

32.4 Early solar burn

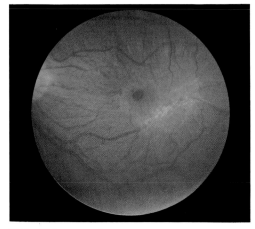

32.2 Hole at macula

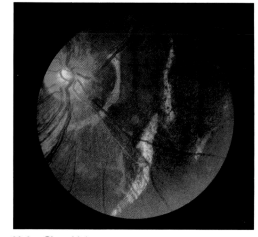

32.3 Choroidal tears

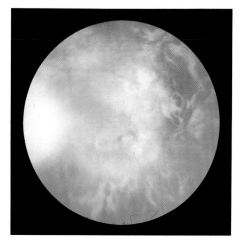

32.5 Intra-ocular metallic foreign body

33 *Neoplasms of the posterior segment*

Pigmented tumours of the choroid constitute the largest group of intra-ocular neoplasms; they may be benign or malignant.

Benign melanoma of the choroid (naevus)

Choroidal naevi occur relatively frequently but are only discovered on ophthalmoscopical examination and do not give rise to symptoms. They appear at the posterior pole of the eye as flat blue or greyish patches, usually about the same size as the disc. The retinal vessels course normally across them and the overlying retina is not raised or detached. This appearance is well illustrated in 33.1A. Fluorescein angiography shows that the lesion masks underlying choroidal fluorescence and shows no tumour circulation (33.1B).

No treatment is required but the patient should be re-examined at intervals, as occasionally a naevus may eventually become the site of a malignant melanoma.

Malignant melanoma of the choroid

Malignant melanoma of the choroid is usually found accidentally during a routine eye examination. Failing that, symptoms are of a retinal detachment and obscuration of the visual field in a particular sector. If, however, the tumour originates at or near the macula, a disturbance of central vision will take place early on.

The tumour starts as a flat infiltration of the choroid, but when it bursts through Bruch's membrane, which separates the choroid from the retina, it grows more freely, pushing the retina before it. 33.2 is a section of an eye containing such a tumour and shows the constriction at the 'neck' of the tumour where it has penetrated Bruch's membrane. If the condition is left untreated the retina becomes completely detached, glaucoma supervenes and extra-ocular extension and metastases occur.

In early cases, before the detachment becomes extensive, the tumour may be seen ophthalmoscopically as shown in 33.3A Fluorescein angiography may be helpful in the diagnosis of malignant melanoma. It frequently shows mixed areas of masking of choroidal fluorescence and abnormal vascular tumour channels within the choroid which fluoresce brilliantly (33.3B). Sometimes the detachment is sufficiently extensive to hide the tumour from view (33.4). The differential diagnosis in such cases can be very difficult. There will be no retinal tear and the usual predisposing features of a simple detachment — myopia or injury — are unlikely to be present. Transillumination of the eye is often helpful and recently radioactive phosphorus has been used to assist in the diagnosis. The ultrasonic findings may be pathognomonic.

The degree of pigmentation of the tumour varies greatly from the so-called leucosarcoma with minimum pigmentation to a darkly pigmented growth, but this feature is of little importance in assessing the degree of malignancy.

Direct extension of the tumour through the channels in the sclera formed by the perforating vessels and nerves occurs relatively early. Extra-ocular metastases may also occur early and may even lead the patient to seek advice before the primary lesion has been noticed. The metastases are blood-borne and do not affect the lymph nodes. The liver is by far the commonest organ affected and as the metastases may not be clinically evident for many years, prognosis is always uncertain.

The prognosis is related to the site and size of the tumour, orbital and metastatic spread, and cell type.

Melanomas can be treated by photocoagulation, radiotherapy (external beam or local plaque therapy) or surgery. The commonest surgical procedure is enucleation, though it may be possible to resect the tumour whilst preserving the eye in selected cases.

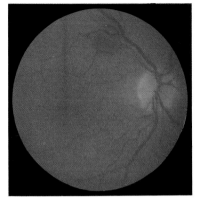

33.1A   Choroidal naevus

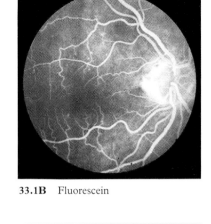

33.1B   Fluorescein

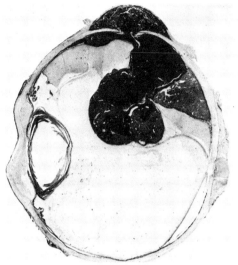

33.2   Section of malignant melanoma

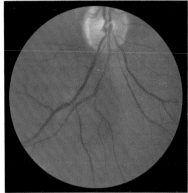

33.3A   Malignant melanoma of choroid

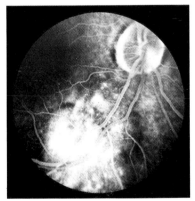

33.3B   Malignant melanoma of choroid
      (fluorescein)

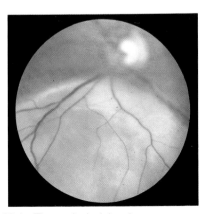

33.4   Tumour/retinal detachment

Neoplasms of the posterior segment *(cont.)*

Retinoblastoma

The pathology of this tumour is of considerable interest. Formerly called a 'glioma' of the retina, it is now recognized as a congenital tumour arising from cell rests of the primitive neuro-ectoderm which form the optic vesicle. One or both eyes are affected and multiple origins of growth are common. It develops most commonly in the first two years of life but a later onset is not unknown.

Retinoblastoma shows a definite hereditary tendency but the mode of transmission is irregular and sporadic cases are in the majority. The risk of a second child of normal parents being affected is about 1%, but the children of an affected parent who has survived the disease show a much higher incidence.

The tumour arises from the inner or outer nuclear layers of the retina and either grows into the vitreous (33.5) or into the subretinal space, causing extensive retinal detachment. In either case the whole vitreous chamber eventually fills with new growth, as seen in 33.6.

As the disease occurs in infants, the first evidence is usually a yellow reflex in the pupil — the so-called 'amaurotic cat's eye' (33.6). The early stages of the tumour are confined to the retina and have a round, pale, elevated appearance (33.7). In the late stages, metastatic nodules appear on the iris and in the anterior chamber.

The differential diagnosis includes congenital abnormalities such as persistence of the primary vitreous, inflammatory conditions and possibly retrolental fibroplasia, although in the latter condition the history of prematurity and oxygen therapy will be obtained.

The growth spreads initially by direct extension through the sclera and along the optic nerve, cerebral involvement being the commonest cause of death. Metastatic spread via the bloodstream does occur but is more common after extra-ocular extension has involved the orbital contents.

Small tumours can be ablated with cryotherapy or photocoagulation. Larger tumours can be treated by radiotherapy using a plaque or external beam source. Enucleation may be necessary if the tumour extends into the optic nerve.

Secondary tumours

The eye is not a common site for metastatic deposits from tumours in other organs of the body, although no doubt small lesions occur in the terminal stages of carcinomatosis but are unnoticed.

If they do occur it is usually in the choroid at the posterior pole, and the breast is the commonest site of the primary lesion. Occasionally the uveal tumour may be the first evidence of the primary lesion, the visual disturbance bringing the patient for advice before the systemic symptoms. Clinically the tumour appears as a circumscribed raised yellowish area at the posterior pole associated with some degree of retinal detachment, as seen in 33.8A. Fluorescein angiography shows much choroidal fluorescence (33.8B). It may spread forward as far as the ciliary body, but rarely penetrates into the vitreous.

Such tumours are part of a generalized carcinomatosis with inevitably a fatal outcome. Radiotherapy and bilateral removal of the suprarenals may secure temporary regression.

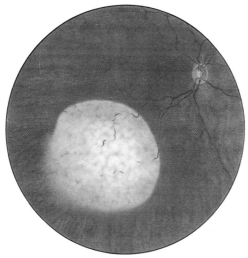

33.5 Large retinoblastoma

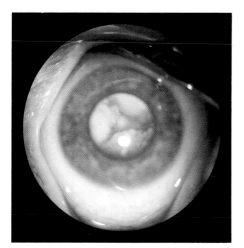

33.6 Amaurotic cat's eye

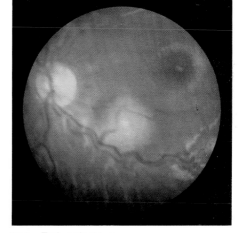

33.7 Early retinoblastoma

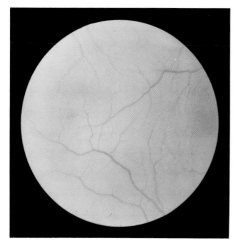

33.8A Typical secondary neoplasm

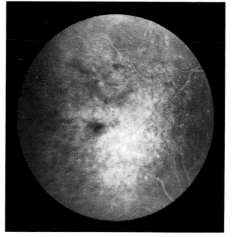

33.8B Typical secondary neoplasm

34 *Retinal detachment*

The pigment epithelium of the retina is firmly adherent to the choroid but only loosely attached to the layer of rods and cones except at the disc and peripherally at the ora serrata. The condition known as retinal detachment is in reality a separation of the main retina from the pigment epithelium, thus re-forming the space originally present in the primary optic vesicle.

The causes of this retinal separation are many and the mechanism involved is often obscure. Detachments secondary to neoplasms or exudative lesions of the choroid, as described in previous sections, are easier to understand than the so-called idiopathic type to be discussed here. The fundamental abnormality is the presence of an area of abnormal attachment of the vitreous to the retina. Movement of the eye, or trauma, cause the vitreous to pull on the retina, thus creating a tear or hole. When this has happened fluid vitreous can pass through the hole and strip the retina off the pigment layer. In some cases it is possible to see a small area of retina suspended in the vitreous over the site of the hole; in others a V-shaped tag of retina is pulled up, giving rise to an 'arrowhead' type of tear as depicted in 34.1. The upper temporal region is the most common site.

Myopia is a common predisposing factor and it has been estimated that two-thirds of all idiopathic detachments occur in myopic eyes. As myopia is usually a bilateral condition it follows that if a detachment has occurred in one eye the other eye is also liable to be affected. The association of detachment with myopia is probably due to the stretching and thinning of the coats of the eye associated with the peripheral degenerative areas and the fluid vitreous so commonly found in shortsighted eyes. Trauma, which may be quite trivial, is a frequent precipitating factor.

The history is often quite typical. The patient notices flashes of light in part of the visual field — usually in the nasal area — due to the adherent vitreous pulling on the retina during movements of the eye. Days or weeks later, when the retina starts to detach, a shadow appears in the field corresponding to the affected region. The lower retina is most likely to be detached as the subretinal fluid sinks by the influence of gravity. Sometimes the patient is not aware of anything wrong until the macular region becomes detached, causing loss of central vision. Ophthalmoscopic examination will reveal an area of the retina which is thrown into folds and has a greyish reflex instead of the clear red of the normal retina. The blood vessels should be carefully examined — they can be seen to follow the retinal folds in the detached area and appear darker than normal and devoid of their central reflex. Slight movements of the eye may elicit corresponding movements of the detached retina.

Some vitreous disturbance is always present and may be sufficiently marked to make examination of the fundus difficult.

It is probable that a hole is present in all cases but it may be very difficult to locate, either because it is at the extreme periphery or because it is hidden in a fold of retina. Sometimes a large arc of retina tears away from the ora serrata, producing a dialysis, as illustrated in 34.2, which contrasts with the 'arrowhead' type of tear having small areas of thinned retina surrounding it, as shown in 34.1. The folding and the greyish reflex with the dark blood vessels are well shown in this fundus photograph.

34.3 shows a retinal detachment secondary to a malignant melanoma which can be seen beneath the detached retina.

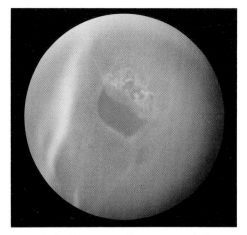

34.1 Retinal tear seen adjacent to mottled retinal degeneration

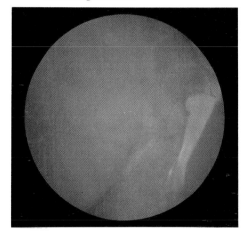

34.2 Retinal detachment with large temporal dialysis

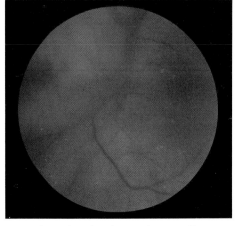

34.3 Secondary detachment due to malignant melanoma

35 *Retinitis pigmentosa*

This interesting retinal condition is a primary degeneration of the neuro-epithelium, accompanied by a widespread pigment disturbance (35.1), narrowing of the vessels and optic atrophy. The aetiology is unknown. The condition is hereditary, although the type of transmission varies and sporadic cases occur in which no family history can be obtained. It is important to attempt to determine the type of transmission in each case so that advice can be given on the likelihood of offspring being affected.

If the disease occurs as a dominant characteristic, half the children of an affected person are likely to exhibit the condition. Consanguinity is an important factor in the incidence of the recessive type. Sex-linkage is common, males exhibiting the fully developed condition, whereas the female carriers who are symptomless may nevertheless show a curious increase in reflection from the fundus, somewhat reminiscent of the tapetal reflex of the cat. Gene probing can identify some carriers of retinitis pigmentosa. Retinitis pigmentosa is the final phenotypic expression of probably a great number of varied inherited defects of rhodopsin metabolism.

Other defects of a degenerative nature may be encountered; thus the association of pigmentary degeneration of the retina with obesity, polydactyly, hypogenitalism and mental retardation constitutes the Laurence-Moon-Biedl syndrome.

The earliest symptom is relative night blindness, which may be first noticed in childhood and is due to the depression of function of the rods, which subserve scotopic vision. The degeneration is bilateral, first affecting the equatorial region and producing a ring scotoma in the visual fields. The scotoma gradually spreads out towards the periphery and in towards fixation, until only a small central field remains. Although the acuity of central vision may be quite good the patient is very severely handicapped by the gross field loss. The remaining visual field typically disappears in middle age, and cataract formation is common. 35.5 is a composite chart of the visual fields showing a typical ring scotoma above, which in the chart below has progressed to leave only a small central area, sometimes described as a 'tubular' field.

The fundus picture is striking in an advanced case. The optic disc is pale and waxy in appearance, the retinal vessels are markedly narrowed and may appear as mere threads. The typical spidery pigment deposits, which have been likened to the Haversian systems in bone, are scattered widely over the peripheral retina. The pigment is frequently found lying along the wall of the veins, as is clearly shown in the fundus photograph (35.2). This migration of pigment from the retinal pigmentary epithelium allows the choroid to be seen more clearly, so that a tessellated pattern and individual choroidal vessels can be seen (35.3).

In an early case the pigment is only present in the equatorial region, while the extreme periphery and central areas appear normal (35.4).

Patients and their families are investigated to confirm the diagnosis and identify the pattern of inheritance so that prognostic and genetic advice can be offered if desired. Electroretinography (ERG), visual fields, family pedigree and ophthalmoscopy aid the diagnosis. Treatment is very disappointing. The disease is subject to remissions which may coincide with some particular therapy, giving rise to false hopes of improvement, but prevention on eugenic lines gives the best hope of eradicating the condition.

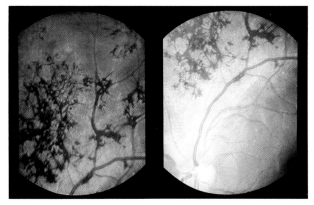

35.1 Typical pigmentary changes

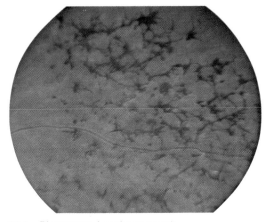

35.2 Pigmentary deposits on vessels

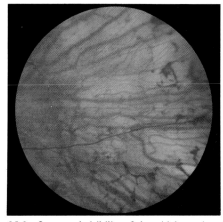

35.3 Increased visibility of choroidal vessels

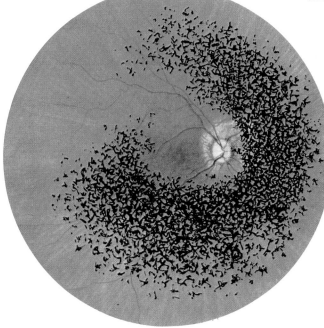

35.4 Localised distribution of pigment

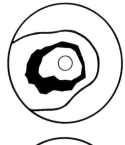

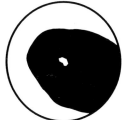

35.5 Typical field defects

36

Heredo-macular degenerations

These diseases have differing inheritance patterns and are all characterized by diminution of central vision. Some are associated with systemic disease, others with disease in other parts of the retina; many tend to be progressive.

Doyne's honeycomb choroiditis/dominant drusen

This is characterized by the appearance of numerous colloid deposits in the pigment epithelium between the optic disc and the macula (even on the nasal side of the disc, 36.1A and fluorescein, 36.1B). The condition is familial, more often seen in women and is usually dominant. As the condition progresses, the deposits increase in size and extent and a disciform macular degeneration may take place leading finally to atrophy of the macular region.

Best's disease/vitelline degeneration

This is a dominant condition occurring in differing age groups starting in the second decade and upwards. It is characterized by progressive loss of central vision. Biomicroscopically there is swelling at the macula and usually there appears to be a deposit of yellowish material underneath the pigment epithelium which becomes elevated like the yolk of an egg (36.2A). Fluorescein angiography at this stage shows pronounced masking of choroidal fluorescence by the lesion but the surrounding retina appears normal (36.2B). With progression of the disease there is reabsorption of the yellow deposit to be replaced by an atrophic scar. During this process a disciform degeneration may occur. The electro-oculogram (EOG) is always reduced in the very early stages of the disease even if the fundus appears normal and the electroretinogram (ERG) remains unaffected.

Bull's eye maculopathy

This includes a whole spectrum of disease: some are confined solely to the macula and others associated with central and peripheral dystrophy of rods and cones. They may be dominant or recessive and may start from the second decade onwards. Biomicroscopically all show a peppery deposit in a bull's eye form at the macula (36.3A). This is demonstrated much better by means of fluorescein angiography (36.3B). One of the commoner conditions with changes outside the macula is Stargardt's or fundus flavimaculatus which shows yellowish flecks surrounding the posterior pole of the retina and the choroid may be dark or light, a feature which is demonstrated even better on fluorescein angiography.

Other hereditary degenerations

Just some of the rarer macular degenerations are mentioned below.

Sorsby's degeneration is a dominant condition characterized by a large disciform degeneration appearing in the fifth decade. There are often yellowish deposits at the fovea prior to the development of the disciform lesion and in half the cases there is peripheral atrophy of the retina. The EOG and ERG are normal.

Pattern dystrophy consists of a number of sub-types where there is pigmentation in bizarre patterns in the macular region. In all cases there is a reduced EOG and the vision is usually quite good considering the physical appearance.

X-linked juvenile retinoschisis may present with diminished central vision as well as the field defect from the schisis. This is due to a very distinctive cystoid type of macular oedema.

Polymorphous dystrophy is dominant, characterised by atrophy of the macula which may originate as a disciform lesion.

Familial lipid degeneration

This condition can be classified according to the age of onset, but the pathology is essentially a primary lipid degeneration of the ganglion cells of the entire nervous system, in which the ganglion cells of the retina are involved.

The most common form of these rare diseases, Tay-Sachs disease (formerly called familial amaurotic idiocy), is typically seen in children of Jewish ancestry. Clinically the child is normal at birth but fails to develop normally and cannot sit or hold its head up, owing to weakness of the muscles of the neck and back. Finally it becomes completely paralysed and dies in a state of marasmus.

The ophthalmoscopic appearance will confirm the diagnosis, as the fundus picture seen in 36.4 is quite typical. It resembles that caused by acute obstruction of the central retinal artery, although the aetiology is altogether different. Around the macula is a white, somewhat raised area fading off into normal fundus at the periphery. At the centre of the white area the fovea shows clearly as a 'cherry-red' spot.

There is no treatment for the condition.

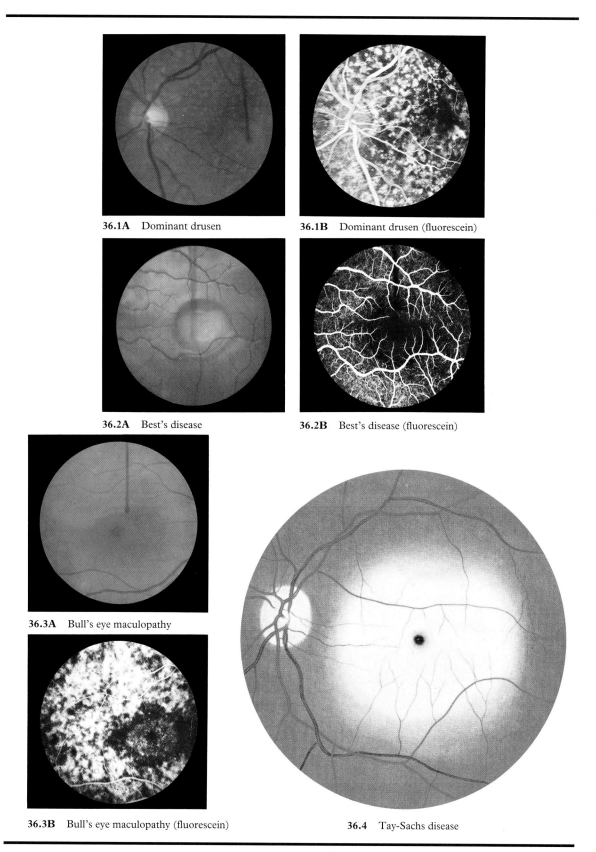

36.1A Dominant drusen

36.1B Dominant drusen (fluorescein)

36.2A Best's disease

36.2B Best's disease (fluorescein)

36.3A Bull's eye maculopathy

36.3B Bull's eye maculopathy (fluorescein)

36.4 Tay-Sachs disease

37 *Senile macular degenerations*

The patient with senile macular degeneration notices gradual or sudden blurring or distortion of vision. The patient may report that straight lines appear distorted, crooked or have gaps. Patients with recent onset of these symptoms should be referred promptly for ophthalmic assessment for a treatable underlying lesion. Senile degeneration of the macula is the commonest cause of blind registration in England and Wales. The central region of vision only is affected and peripheral vision remains good.

Drusen or colloid bodies

Small well defined yellowish spots are commonly found at the posterior pole in elderly patients. They are well illustrated in 37.1 and are due to deposition of hyaline material on Bruch's membrane. Fortunately they cause little visual disturbance in themselves. Fluorescein angiography shows them as bright spots of choroidal windowing appearing early in the dye transit and showing no late leakage. In many cases they are a precursor of macular degeneration.

Exudative or disciform macular degeneration

This condition is associated with diminution of central vision which may be rapid or slow in onset. There is a raised area of retina lying at the macula which is usually surrounded with drusen. The disciform swelling may be caused by a simple pigment epithelial detachment or a neovascular membrane or both.

Pigment epithelial detachments present as elevations of the pigment epithelium with or without an overlying serous retinal detachment. Fluorescein angiography shows slow delineation of the pigment epithelial detachment with dye but later there is intensification throughout the whole area (37.3A & B). The benefit of laser treatment of retinal pigment epithelial detachments is questionable.

Neovascular disciforms are usually more severe and rapid in onset than the above. Biomicroscopy shows a serous neuroretinal detachment with underlying pigment epithelial detachment or degeneration. There is frequently subretinal haemorrhage, hard exudate surrounding the macula and a dark central ring at the level of the pigment epithelium which represents the neovascular membrane (37.4A). Fluorescein angiography demonstrates the neovascular membrane elegantly at an early stage of dye transit (37.4B). There is rapid leakage from the new vessels into the surrounding pigment epithelium. Pathologically these changes represent a breakdown in Bruch's membrane with degenerative changes in the overlying pigment epithelium. Through this grow new vessels derived from the veins in the choroid. They proliferate under the pigment epithelium and frequently bleed which may be so severe as to cause a large subretinal haemorrhage or even burst through the retina into the vitreous. Laser treatment may be suitable in some cases.

Atrophic macular degeneration

Dry atrophic macular degeneration is an atrophy where there is a minimal elevation of neuroretina and pigment epithelium with degeneration of these tissues and the underlying choroid to varying degrees (37.2). Central vision is naturally severely impaired and is usually of gradual onset. Some of these cases probably represent a burned-out, scarred neovascular disciform degeneration but in others a more insidious atrophic process seems to occur. Fluorescein angiography shows marked windowing of underlying choroid and also delineates choroidal sclerosis. There is no treatment for these cases.

Treatment of senile macular degeneration

All these conditions tend to be bilateral with one eye presenting at varying times before the other. It is important in unilateral cases to warn patients to seek help immediately there is any distortion or diminution of vision in the other eye. Laser is of questionable benefit in atrophic senile macular degeneration and retinal pigment epithelial detachments. Laser can be used to ablate neovascular membranes to stabilise vision. Laser does not usually restore vision which has already been lost, and neovascular membranes have a high recurrence rate after laser ablation. When laser treatment is ineffective it is important to register the patient as visually impaired and to try varying types of visual aid to improve their central visual acuity. The patient's peripheral vision is preserved in senile macular degeneration.

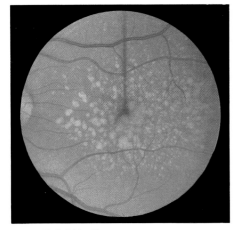

37.1 Colloid bodies

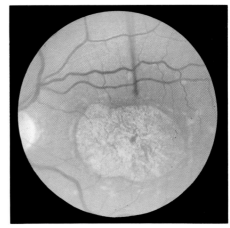

37.2 Atrophic macular degeneration

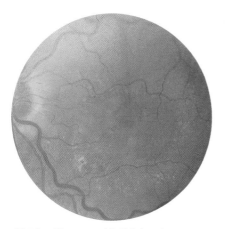

37.3A Pigment epithelial detachment

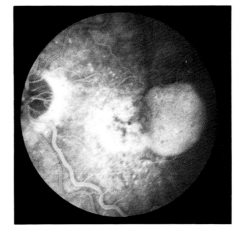

37.3B Pigment epithelial detachment

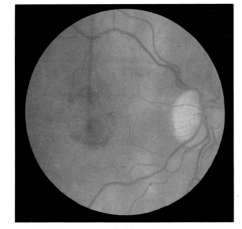

37.4A Neovascular disciform lesion

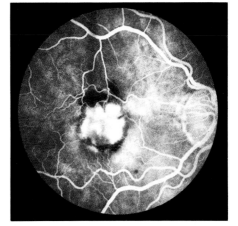

37.4B Neovascular disciform lesion (fluorescein)

38 *Miscellaneous fundus conditions*

These are a recently recognized group of disorders with the bulk of visible damage falling upon the pigment epithelium. In many it is not sure if the pigment epithelium is the primary source of pathology or if it is due to changes in the small underlying vessels of the choroid.

Central serous retinopathy

This is a strange condition probably encompassing several different types of pathogenesis, but best included in this section. It is characterized by a serous neuroretinal detachment in the macular region (38.1A). It occurs chiefly in young adults and between the 30s and 50s (predominantly in males). Symptoms are blurred central vision, a varying degree of distortion and micropsia. Fluorescein angiography may show an isolated focal leak of dye early on from the pigment epithelium which progresses to give a smoke stack appearance (38.1B & C) or on the other hand may show several areas of choroidal windowing and fluorescein leakage. The natural history in younger patients is for spontaneous resolution within a few months but in chronic cases, particularly in those in the 40–50 age group it may be beneficial to treat the areas of focal leakage with Argon laser provided they do not underlie the macula.

Krill's pigment epitheliopathy

This mimics central serous retinopathy in symptoms and occurs in a similar young age group of 20–40. The disease is usually more insidious in onset and resolves well without treatment. The appearance on biomicroscopy is of slight elevation of the neuroretina at the macula with some brown and deep red underlying swellings (38.2A). Fluorescein angiography may show some granular areas of choroidal transmission defects underlying the macula (38.2B) or no abnormality at all.

Multiplacoid epitheliopathy

This is usually an acute condition causing diminution of central vision and is sometimes bilateral. Biomicroscopically it shows as a large serous retinal detachment with underlying small areas of pallor and swelling of the pigment epithelium (38.3A).

Fluorescein angiography in the acute phase shows areas of profound masking of choroidal fluorescence which correspond to the pigment epithelial lesions and in the convalescent phase these areas begin to atrophy and show pronounced choroidal windowing with leakage of dye (38.3B). The aetiology is obscure but many patients have had preceding acute viral-type illness or a course of systemic antibiotics. Treatment is unsatisfactory.

Geographic pigment epitheliopathy

This is a very slow chronic disease, again usually bilateral. It is characterised by progressive visual loss centrally and appears as a serpiginous or geographic pattern of pigment epithelial loss and atrophy (38.4A). Fluorescein angiography demonstrates these areas very nicely with new lesions masking choroidal fluorescence but later atrophy leading to pronounced choroidal windowing (38.4B). The evolution of the lesions seems to be from isolated small areas of pigment epithelial disease which later coalesce with newer and older lesions.

Vogt Koyanagi Harada disease

This is a strange condition rather similar to placoid epitheliopathy but there tends to be a more massive exudative retinal detachment. It is commoner in the East. It causes severe loss of central vision and may be accompanied by an iritis and signs of meningism. Biomicroscopy shows usually a large exudative retinal detachment with underlying areas of swollen pale pigment epithelium. Fluorescein angiography in the active phase shows areas of masking corresponding to these pigment epithelial lesions which later on leak fluorescein. As the acute phase passes the pigment epithelium shows many areas of atrophy, the exudative detachment tends to settle and the fluorescein angiogram shows much choroidal windowing with little late leakage of dye. In the later stages of the disease there is often depigmentation of lids, skin and lashes causing poliosis and vitiligo. Treatment seems to be best with an initial high dose of systemic steroid rapidly tapering off.

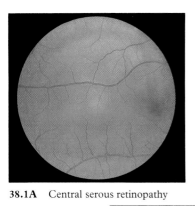
38.1A Central serous retinopathy

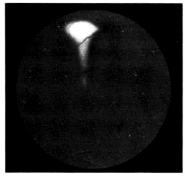
38.1B Central serous retinopathy

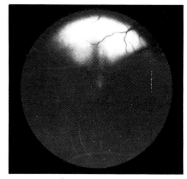
38.1C Central serous retinopathy

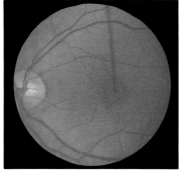
38.2A Krill's retinopathy

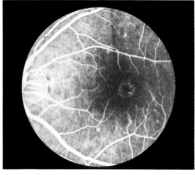
38.2B Krill's retinopathy

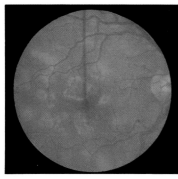
38.3A Multiplacoid epitheliopathy

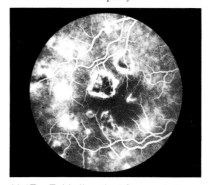
38.3B Epitheliopathy (fluorescein)

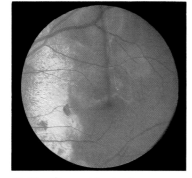
38.4A Geographic atrophy

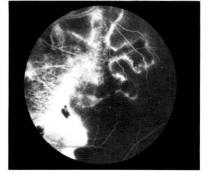
38.4B Geographic atrophy

39 *Ophthalmic HIV*

The majority of patients with AIDS will have some form of ophthalmic involvement at some stage of their disease. These ophthalmic manifestations fall into four general categories: retinal vasculitis, opportunistic infections, ocular and adnexal tumours, and neuro-ophthalmic disease. Retinal vasculitis may also be seen in asymptomatic HIV positive patients who do not have AIDS.

Retinal vasculitis

Here the patient has cotton wool spots, retinal haemorrhages or microaneurysms indicative of retinal capillary disease (39.1). There may be signs of macular or optic nerve ischaemia.

Opportunist infections

One of the most striking manifestations of ocular AIDS is opportunist retinitis caused by a wide range of intracellular infections, including Cytomegalovirus (39.2), Herpes simplex, *Toxoplasma gondii* and *Candida albicans.* Conjunctivitis and keratitis due to 'conventional' organisms is seen with increased frequency in patients with AIDS.

AIDS associated tumours

Kaposi's sarcoma involving the eyelids or conjunctiva may be the presenting symptom of AIDS (39.3), as may orbital lymphoma.

Neuro-ophthalmic manifestations of AIDS

Visual field defects, strabismus and papilloedema may all be caused by AIDS. These manifestations follow central nervous system opportunist infections, neoplasms or HIV associated demyelination.

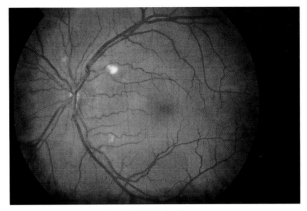

39.1 Retinal vasculitis in HIV infection

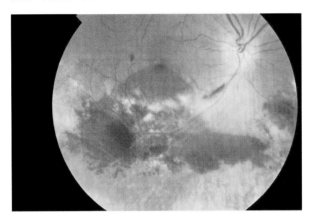

39.2 Cytomegalovirus retinitis

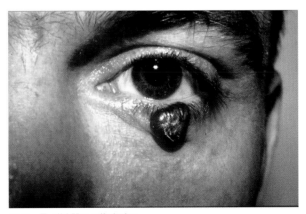

39.3 Eyelid Kaposi's lesion

40 *Assessing loss of vision and painful eyes*

The painful red eye for the primary physician

The assessment of any patient with painful red eye(s) requires a careful assessment by history, measurement of visual acuity and ocular examination. This chapter is aimed at helping the primary physician to diagnose the commoner causes of a painful red eye when a slit lamp microscope is not available. The conditions are all illustrated elsewhere in the text.

Painful conditions of the lid and conjunctiva

The sensation of a foreign body in the eye accompanies infective and allergic conjunctivititis, blepharitis, lid and lash malposition, corneal abrasion, keratitis, and of course, foreign bodies. The presence of a discharge suggests conjunctivitis and the history may further suggest the likely type.

A short history and a purulent discharge occurs in bacterial conjunctivitis whilst a clear discharge is typical of a viral or allergic conjunctivitis. An atopic history frequently accompanies allergic conjunctivitis whilst a long history of low grade irritation with crusts on the lashes suggests blepharoconjunctivititis.

The acuity should be measured in each eye. The position of the lids and lashes are noted and the lid margin is inspected for signs of blepharitis and cysts. The conjunctiva is inspected for the pattern of injection and the lids are everted to look for foreign bodies. Fluorescein is instilled to exclude corneal epithelial defects. The cornea should be bright and clear and the iris details should be readily visible in both eyes if the patient has simple conjunctivitis or blepharitis. There are several findings which exclude the diagnosis of simple blepharitis or conjunctivitis. A drop in visual acuity suggests an alternative diagnosis. A history of photophobia and aching painful red eye should immediately alert the clinician to the possibility of uveitis or keratitis, as should a previous history of these conditions.

Painful conditions of the cornea

Corneal erosions are frequently seen in patients who wear their contact lenses too long, or following ultraviolet keratitis from sunbeds or welding. Keratitis sicca is a common cause of corneal erosions in elderly patients and in patients with connective tissue diseases.

Corneal abrasions are painful and there is often a history of a foreign body entering the eye. Abrasions and erosions stain with a solution of fluorescein and are treated by padding and prophylactic topical antibiotic. Analgesics are prescribed symptomatically and a topical cycloplegic, such as a single drop of homatropine, also helps to ease the pain.

Infective keratitis usually complicates some local abnormality of the ocular surface rather than occurring as an isolated entity. Contact lens wear, corneal abrasion, dry eyes and previous keratitis all increase the risk of developing this condition. Careful examination reveals a white corneal infiltrate. It is often easier to examine the cornea after instilling topical anaesthetic. Patients with keratitis should be referred urgently to an ophthalmologist for specialist investigation and management.

Uveitis

Acute anterior uveitis causes a deep ache (rather than foreign body sensation) and photophobia. The patient may give a history of previous uveitis or of a systemic condition which is associated with uveitis.

The visual acuity is frequently reduced. Iris details are obscured by anterior chamber inflammation in marked cases. The pain is not alleviated by topical anaesthetic drops. Anterior uveitis is treated by local steroid and mydriatic in the first instance. The primary physician should withold such treatment and seek urgent ophthalmic opinion if uncertain about the diagnosis or if there are any features which suggest acute glaucoma (see below). All patients with anterior uveitis need ophthalmic referral to confirm the diagnosis and identify occult secondary glaucoma and posterior uveitis.

Acute glaucoma

Acute glaucoma causes intense pain and a reduction in vision and frequently occurs in the elderly and hypermetropes. The patient often vomits because of the intensity of the pain and she (or he) notes haloes surrounding bright lights because of corneal oedema. Iris details are obscured by corneal oedema and the anterior chamber is shallow.

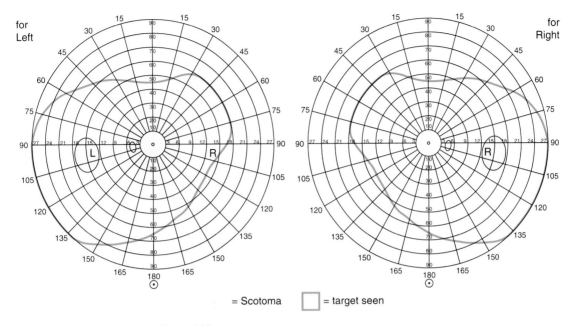

= Scotoma   □ = target seen

40.1 Left central scotoma (optic neuritis)

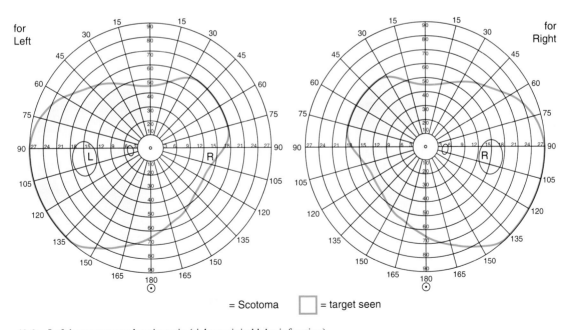

= Scotoma   □ = target seen

40.2 Left homonymous hemianopia (right occipital lobe infarction)

Acute glaucoma is treated in the first instance with miotics and oral ocular hypotensive medication. Treatment should be given by an ophthalmologist and urgent referral is indicated. It is important not to mis-diagnose a case of acute glaucoma. Delayed treatment or inadvertent treatment with a mydriatic worsens the prognosis.

Less common causes of a painful red eye

Orbital cellulitis and dysthyroid eye disease are dis-cussed in Chapter 2. Scleritis and episcleritis are discussed in Chapter 14.

Visual loss

This section is aimed at helping the primary physician to diagnose the commoner causes of visual loss. All patients with visual loss require a careful history, mea-surement of visual acuity and fields and ocular examination.

Painless gradual loss of vision

The commonest causes are refractive errors, cataract, glaucoma, macular degeneration and diabetic eye disease. Enquiry may reveal a personal or family history of these conditions.

The acuity is measured by asking the patient to read the letters on a chart from the correct distance using each eye in turn. The vision improves when the patient looks through a pinhole in refractive errors less than about four dioptres. The visual fields tested by confrontation may yield useful information about hemianopias and other gross visual field defects. Subtle field defects, such as those of early glaucoma, are best detected by formal perimetry. Some common visual field defects are illustrated (40.1–40.3).

The red reflex is examined by looking through an ophthalmoscope held at one metre from the patient's pupil. Cataracts show up as shadows against the red reflex, or prevent the red reflex from being seen. The ophthalmoscope is now held close to the patient to examine the lens and optic disc. Cupping of the optic disc suggests the patient may have glaucoma. In most cases it is not possible to view the entire macula satis-factorily without using mydriatic drops[1]. The fundus is examined, looking particularly for signs of macular degeneration or diabetic retinopathy.

Painful acute loss of vision

The commonest causes of painful acute visual loss are uveitis, keratitis and acute glaucoma. The diagnosis of the painful red eye has already been discussed above.

Retrobulbar neuritis is usually painful and the patient complains of uniocular visual loss and ache on eye movement. The patient frequently reports that colours seem faded or that the central portion of the visual field is missing. There is a drop in visual acuity, loss of colour vision and the patient has a central scotoma. Pupillary testing shows relative loss of the consensual light response. The optic disc may look normal initially but becomes pale after several weeks. It is important to refer patients with suspected optic neuropathy to confirm the diagnosis and exclude compressive optic neuropathy.

Painless acute loss of vision

The commonest causes of painless acute visual loss are vitreous haemorrhage, retinal vascular occlusions, retinal detachment, acute macular degeneration, optic neuropathy and cerebrovascular disease. It may be necessary to dilate the pupil to diagnose these condi-tions unless visual fields have revealed an obvious homonymous hemianopia.

Giant cell arteritis typically presents in an elderly patient with headaches, malaise and muscular weak-ness. Giant cell arteritic ischaemic optic neuropathy is painless, but is frequently associated with headache. There is profound sudden uniocular drop in vision and pupillary testing shows relative loss of the consen-sual light response[2]. The optic disc is swollen. The erythrocyte sedimentation rate is markedly elevated. It is important to give high dose steroids to prevent blindness in the other eye, myocardial infarction or stroke. The diagnosis is best confirmed histologically by temporal artery biopsy.

[1]Mydriatic drops may rarely precipitate acute glaucoma in patients with shallow anterior chambers. These patients are usually hypermetropic, and the iris can be seen to be close to the cornea when a light is shone on the eye from the side.

[2]Relative loss of the consensual light reflex is demonstrated by the constriction of both when light is shone at the normal eye and dilation of both pupils when light is then rapidly transferred to the affected eye.

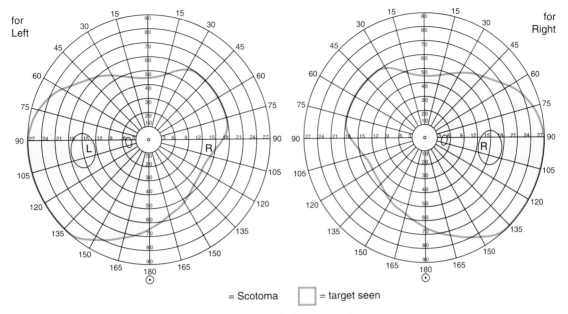

= Scotoma   = target seen

40.3 Bitemporal hemianopia (chiasmal compression by pituitary tumour)

Index